Total Health
and
Food Power

Total Health and Food Power

*Principles of Healthful Living
and Outstanding Vegetarian Recipes from
Glendale Adventist Medical Center*

by

Rose Budd Ludlow, M.A., R.D.

*Consulting Dietitian
Formerly, Director of Dietary Service
Glendale Adventist Medical Center
Glendale, California*

*Millions suffer sickness and infirmities because
they fail to know and use commonsense principles of health.*

Published by

Woodbridge Press / Santa Barbara, California

Published and distributed by

Woodbridge Press Publishing Company
Post Office Box 6189
Santa Barbara, California 93160

Printed in the United States of America
Distributed simultaneously in Canada

Library of Congress Cataloging-in-Publication Data

Ludlow, Rose Budd.
  Total health and food power.

  1. Low-calorie diet—Recipes. 2. Health.
3. Nutrition. 4. Vegetarian cookery. 5. Diet
therapy. I. Title.
RM222.2.L73 1985   641.5'63   85-29594
ISBN 0-88007-158-3

Photographic credits: front cover, Loma Linda University Medical Center; back
  cover, top, Elwyn Spaulding; bottom, Tomatis Alain.

Illustrations: Linda Trujillo

Dedication

This book is dedicated to our dear friends, Alfred and Evelyn Montapert, whose love and wisdom supported me through my writing. May the principles outlined in this volume be a constant guide for the seeker after the truth.

Acknowledgments

This book is offered as a guide to total health and optimal living. It is my hope that it may prove a useful reference in incorporating healthful practice in everyday living.

I am indebted to those who provided the inspiration and dedication that made this volume possible, including my husband, Bradley, and my sister, Naomi Parson.

To Alfred Montapert, an eminently successful businessman, particular acknowledgment is gratefully made for the assistance given in finance, inspiration, and direction. Sincere appreciation is extended to Blanche Bobbitt, Ph.D., for her careful, efficient editing of the entire manuscript; to Kathleen Zolber, Ph.D., for her valuable suggestions to the finished manuscript; to Charles Strachan, M.D., and Richard Thorp, M.D., for reviewing Chapters 12 and 13 respectively; and to Don Jacobsen, D.Min., and Hayward Shaffer, M.A., for reviewing Chapters 16 and 17.

The following dietitians calculated the amounts of nutrients listed with each recipe: Grace Ogura, M.S., R.D.; Enid O'Young, M.S., R.D.; Cindy Hudson, R.D.; Betty Eaton, R.D.; Monika Bilinski, R.D.; Alma Gepford, R.D.; Shirley Gumbao, B.S., Winna Chen, R.D.; and Joy Atiga, R.D.

Recognition is due also to Sammie Johannes, a successful chef, and Henry Wakeam, an accomplished baker, for the recipes they provided.

To each and every one of the above contributors I express heartfelt thanks.

The Author

Contents

Section I: *Principles of Healthful Living*

Section II: *Recipes*

Section I: Principles of Healthful Living

Welcome to an Adventure in Health

Dear Reader,

When the deluge of health and weight control books on the market overwhelms you, take a break—refresh yourself! Then come back and read *Nature's* proven way to *Total Health and Food Power*.

My lifetime work has focused on *Total Health and Food Power*. Here are techniques and formulas I have learned that have proven to be beneficial to the health and well-being of many, many people.

Quality of life is improved by daily practices that contribute to the prevention of illness and disease. Money is wisely spent on fresh air and sunshine, on gardens and vegetables, on orchards and fruits, on exercise and adequate diets.

Health is our greatest asset—a precious possession. Without *Health,* pleasures, wisdom, love, life are unfulfilled. *Health* must be earned and pursued through exercise, diet, attitude, discipline, self-control.

The greatest gift in life is life itself. Today people are becoming concerned with the quality of life. The basis of a quality life is optimal health. The decision rests with you to make your life healthy, vigorous, and fulfilled.

Eat to be a winner! Read on . . .

Rose Budd Ludlow, M.A., R.D.
Nutrition Counselor

Why I Wrote This Book

For many years, I have worked with hundreds of people who had lost their health and were seeking help. I have met folks who seemingly had burned themselves out by lifelong careless eating habits. When they could no longer manage, they would enter a hospital with a variety of complications requiring surgery or special treatment. The physcans and dietitians had the responsibility to unite their energies and resources to save lives.

One special serious case comes to mind. A doctor called me one afternoon and asked me to see a patient and try to persuade her to eat. He said unless the patient ate something and kept it down, she could be dead by morning.

The patient had a unique metabolic complication and was unable to retain the food she ate. I visited her and urged her to try something special that I would make for her, explaining that I wished her to eat a small amount of food every two hours—all night. She resisted, but I explained that I was there to help her and I was going to attend to her needs all through the night. The experience was rewarding and exciting. When the doctor visited her the next morning, he couldn't believe what had been accomplished. The patient was alive—and she improved slowly during the next two weeks and was discharged.

Physicians and dietitians working closely together can achieve remarkable results. I have been convinced for years that many of the problems of hospital patients are the result of wrong living habits, inadequate eating practices, and incorrect choices. Why not make some changes that will ensure a long, happy life? Knowledge is essential to make wise choices. Changes in life-style that may be necessary for health are not always easy to accomplish.

I have held many weight management clinics and have met hundreds of people who could benefit from classes, clinics, and consultation in nutrition or from additional nutritional information and recipes to make their life-style meet their needs.

Changing life-styles and habits is not easy unless one is convinced of a real need to do so. I recall a patient who came to me for diabetic instruction. His doctor had explained that a special diet was needed to cope with this disease. With illustrative materials, I began instructing him about the various foods that he could or could not tolerate, but I seemed to receive much resistance. I had two lists of foods that I was attempting to show him. On the first list were foods he could eat without restriction. The second list consisted of foods to be restricted or eliminated. One of the items to be eliminated was alcohol. I no sooner mentioned the word "alcohol" than he became so angry that he called out, "Lady, if you think I will give up my highballs, you have another think coming."

I was convinced by now that he was not learning and that my efforts were futile. So I closed my book and started to put away my materials. This act shocked him. He apologized and begged me to continue. He was willing now and ready to listen. From there on he was most attentive and probably one of the best students I ever had. When we were finished, he thanked me and asked me if I would kindly repeat the instructions for his wife so she could cook properly for him. Incidentally, when I took his diet history, his daily food pattern was as follows: for breakfast, a cup of coffee and a doughnut; for lunch, a hamburger and coffee; and dinner was a big T-bone steak and a highball. There were no fruits, vegetables, grains, or cereals in his diet pattern. I asked him where were the vitamins, minerals, and other nutrients he needed?

One week later, he returned with his wife, eager for her to learn all about the recommended diet. After the introduction, he excused himself to care for the children so his wife could learn with undivided attention. As soon as he was out of the room, she turned to me and asked, "What did you say to my husband last week? You must have scared him to death because he has not had a drink since you talked with him." I explained the diet pattern and she understood the importance of following the plan as presented. The patient was ready and willing to follow the new dietary regime when he realized his life depended on it.

Many people have less stressful situations than the one just described. However, everyone needs to have a plan for optimal living. By making a plan, the chances are increased for reaching desired goals. People need to think through just what they want in life, what they want healthwise. The first step is to make up one's mind, then to pursue the plan diligently to achieve success.

Because of the many requests for dietary information and healthful recipes, I was motivated to write this book. My friends urged me to share the "secrets" of my own success in healthful living. This volume will provide such information.

Although clinical diagnostic information will not be included, a new discipline for obtaining an adequate nutritional intake will be discussed. Since we are what we eat, this volume will provide information regarding intelligent choices. Everyone must choose what is best for him, and each must live with the choices he makes.

The problems of caloric intake versus caloric expenditure will also be considered. And, since exercise is an important part of total health, some suggestions as to how much and what kind of exercise will be included. In addition, the vegetarian diet and the art of vegetable cookery will be presented.

Since heart disease is the number one killer, consideration will be given to ways to avoid or delay onset of this disease by controlling the diet. A chapter dealing with foods considered an integral part of reducing the risk of cancer is also included. Another chapter will deal with stress, and there is also a chapter on depression and how to deal with it.

As the various phases of nutrition are explored, I hope the reader will conclude that nutrition is an integral aspect of life both for the individual and the family.

Chapter 1

Nutrition Is the Key to Total Health

"You are what you eat" has been said many times, many ways. The purpose of this chapter is to impress upon the reader the importance of practicing intelligent eating habits.

The American people are possibly the most inadequately fed Nation in the world, not because of the unavailability of food or the economy of the Nation, but rather because of the abundance of refined foods and the hit-or-miss choices made regarding what is consumed.

For example, breakfast should be a nourishing meal to prepare the body for activities of the day. Instead, breakfast is often neglected or overlooked completely.

There is an abundance of misinformation to add to the confusion. Fad diets of one kind or another do not contribute to intelligent food practices. On the contrary, fad diets, if followed for any length of time, can be devastating.

Snacking and eating between meals should be avoided. This habit impairs adequate nutrition. Often one is not hungry at mealtime, so eats only a snack. Snacks are usually made up of excessive "empty" calories with negligible nutrition. To the overweight, perhaps, "empty calories" sound like just what is needed! But are they? The answer is that empty calories usually are fattening; that is, they are empty only of nutrients! Some foods that provide so-called empty calories include candy, cakes, pies, chips, and sodas. Foods with so-called empty calories are often classified as "junk" foods!

Adequate nutrition requires the daily intake of nutrients from the following five categories:

Proteins are so important that without them life cannot exist. Proteins are the major constituents of body tissues and are by far the largest and most complex of molecules, made up of more than twenty different amino acids. They are compounds containing carbon, hydrogen, oxygen, and nitrogen. Proteins are changed by enzymes in the body to amino acids. Proteins may be complete or incomplete. If complete, they contain the eight "essential" amino acids—the ones the body needs but cannot itself produce. The body can make proteins and build cells if all the essential amino acids are present. Body proteins wear out and must be replaced. Therefore, the right protein foods must be eaten to meet the body's need.

Sources of "complete" proteins are meat, fish, poultry, milk, cheese, eggs, soybeans.

Sources of "incomplete" proteins are corn, cereals, grains, nuts, and legumes, including beans, lentils, garbanzos, and split peas. Because each of these may contain amino acids others lack, by simple combinations such as beans with corn, one has a complete protein. Other combinations include cereal with milk, or legumes with peanut butter.

Carbohydrates are compounds containing carbon, hydrogen, and oxygen. They include the sugars and starches in the diet that are a source of energy. Carbohydrates are changed by enzymes in the body to the simple sugars glucose and fructose, which circulate to all parts of the body via the blood stream and pass from the blood stream into the tissues and cells by way of the fluids which surround the cells. Carbohydrates are needed not only for body energy, but also for the digestion of fats. When the body has carbohydrates available as energy "fuel," it is less likely to use up protein as an energy source.

Too often an excessive amount of carbohydrates is included in the daily diet and, as a consequence, many problems result. Too many sugars and starches can be the source of problems such as dental cavities, heart attacks, diabetes onset, hyperglycemia, obesity. The body needs can be satisfied with such carbohydrate sources as fruits, vegetables, grains, cereals.

Fats are compounds containing carbon, hydrogen, and oxygen, and may be "solid" (saturated) or "liquid" (unsaturated). The unsaturated fats have fewer hydrogen atoms than the saturated—monounsaturated lacking 2 hydrogen atoms, and polyunsaturated lacking 4 or more hydrogen atoms.

Fats are necessary for fuel, to insulate the body, to maintain constant body temperature, to carry fat-soluble vitamins that aid in the utilization of carbohydrates and proteins, to promote normal growth. But fats are needed only in small quantities.

The kinds of fats chosen are extremely important to health. Solid animal or saturated fat (hard fat) should be minimized in preference to oil of vegetable origin with little or no saturation. Furthermore, margarines from such sources as the soybean, safflower, corn, or olive should be used instead of butter. While fats are needed in the diet for many reasons, the amount and kind used should be carefully considered.

Vitamins have an essential role in maintaining health. In fact, the human body cannot exist without them. Most are readily available in the usual food consumed.

The fat-soluble vitamins are A, D, E, and K. Sources of vitamin A are cantaloupe, apricots, green and yellow vegetables, margarine, cream, and egg yolk. Vitamin A is gradually destroyed by exposure to air and heat. A deficiency of vitamin A may cause night blindness or other problems.

Sources of vitamin D are egg yolks, dairy products, corn oil. This vitamin is stable to heat, age, and storage. Its main function is to aid in calcium and phosphorous absorption and metabolism. A deficiency of vitamin D may cause rickets, soft bones, poor teeth, and skeletal deformities.

Sources of vitamin E are wheat germ, leafy vegetables, vegetable oils, egg yolks, legumes, peanuts, and margarine. This vitamin is stable to all methods of food processing; however, it is destroyed by rancidity. One purpose of vitamin E is to maintain the function of reproductive and muscular tissues.

Sources of vitamin K are cabbage, cauliflower, spinach, and other leafy vegetables; soybean oil and other vegetable oils. Vitamin K is stable to heat, light, and exposure to air. The chief function of vitamin K is to aid in the formation of prothrombin and the clotting of blood.

The water-soluble vitamins are B_1, B_2, B_3, B_6, B_9, B_{12}, pantothenic acid, biotin, and C.

Vitamin B_1, thiamine, occurs in whole grains, eggs, nuts, meat, green peas, and potatoes. Thiamine is necessary for carbohydrate metabolism and for regulation of nerves.

Vitamin B_2, riboflavin, occurs in milk, yeast, nuts, meat, dark-green leafy vegetables, mushrooms, and cereals. Riboflavin is necessary for releasing energy from proteins, carbohydrates, and fats to the body cells. B_2 helps also in maintaining mucous membranes.

Vitamin B_3, niacin, occurs in meat, fish, poultry, nuts, whole grains, yeast, and legumes. Niacin assists in the digestion of carbohydrates and proteins.

Vitamin B_6, pyridoxine, occurs in yeast, grains, meat, bananas, and potatoes. Pyridoxine is important in the digestion of proteins and fats.

Vitamin B_9, folic acid, occurs in organ meats, dark-green leafy vegetables, asparagus, milk, and eggs. Folic acid is necessary for blood formation and the digestion of proteins.

Vitamin B_{12}, cobalamine, occurs in milk and eggs. Cobalamine is necessary for the digestion of protein and for the formation of red blood cells.

Pantothenic acid occurs in eggs, organ meats, yeast, milk, legumes, broccoli, kale, sweet potatoes, and yellow corn. Pantothenic acid is necessary for the digestion of carbohydrates, proteins, and fats, and aids in the formation of hormones and nerve-regulating substances.

Biotin occurs in eggs, yeast, organ meats, tomatoes, peanuts, mushrooms, dark-green vegetables, and green beans. Biotin is necessary for the digestion of carbohydrates and fats, and has an important role in several enzyme systems.

Vitamin C, ascorbic acid, occurs in fresh fruits and vegetables such as citrus, tomatoes, broccoli, and cantaloupe. Ascorbic acid is important in the health of bones, teeth, and blood vessels.

Minerals also have an important role in maintaining health. They regulate body fluids, form teeth and bones, participate in the life processes of cells, and are involved in many chemical reactions.

Iron occurs in liver, lean meat, legumes, whole grains, dark-green vegetables, eggs, and dark molasses. Iron is a component of hemoglobin and enzymes involved in the digestion of proteins, fats, and carbohydrates.

Calcium occurs in milk, turnips, green vegetables, clams, oysters, shrimp, salmon. Calcium is important as a major building material for bones and teeth. Many people suffer from osteoporosis caused by a shortage of calcium. The skeleton alone holds about 98 percent of the body's calcium, and the teeth one percent. The remaining one percent is used throughout the body for the regulation of muscles, especially the heart. Calcium is important in clotting blood, nourishing cells, releasing energy, and transmitting nerve impulses. Hence, calcium is one of the most important minerals for the body.

Phosphorus occurs in meat, fish, poultry, milk, cheese, whole grains, legumes. Phosphorus, an important nutritional co-worker of calcium, is found mainly in the bones and teeth. Phosphorus helps to release energy from fats and carbohydrates.

Magnesium occurs in whole grains, nuts, beans, leafy vegetables, and milk. Magnesium is important for bone structure, nerve and muscle activity, release of energy, regulation of body temperature, and fat metabolism.

Sodium, potassium, and chloride are the regulators of the body fluids. Sodium occurs in table salt, salted foods, and most protein foods. Potassium occurs in almost all foods, especially fruits such as bananas, oranges, dates. It may be obtained also from nuts, dry beans, and winter squash. Chloride is supplied almost entirely by sodium chloride commonly known as table salt.

Manganese occurs in nuts, whole grains, vegetables, and fruits. Manganese is needed for reproduction, growth, and normal bone structure.

Copper occurs in organ meats, shellfish, dried legumes, nuts, and cocoa. Copper is needed in the development of red blood cells and respiratory enzymes.

Fluoride occurs in fluoridated water, canned fish, and tea. Fluoride is needed for the formation and strength of teeth and bones.

Zinc occurs in fish, meat, egg yolk, and milk. Zinc is needed for growth, appetite, and digestion. Zinc is also used as a part of many enzymes in the body.

Iodine occurs in seafood and iodized salt. Since a small amount is used by the food-processing industry to disinfect equipment, some of the iodine enters the food chain.

All of the above five categories of nutrients, (proteins, carbohydrates, fats, vitamins, and minerals) may be obtained in the daily diet by planning meals that include foods from the familiar Basic Four Food Groups. These will be discussed in the following chapter on meal planning.

Chapter 2

Meal Planning for the Entire Day

Meals should be planned to include fresh, wholesome food that has been prepared in such a way as to maintain maximum nutritional value. According to a report from the United States Department of Agriculture, a large percent of America's population eat nutritionally inadequate diets not because they are poverty-stricken but because they lack the knowledge and willpower to plan and follow an intelligent, well-balanced nutritional eating pattern. What is such a pattern?

A helpful guide is the familiar Basic Four Food Groups. These food groups are:

1. *Milk group and dairy products:* milk, skim milk, buttermilk, cheese.
2. *Protein group:* eggs, meat, fish, poultry, nuts, legumes, meat alternates.
3. *Fruits and vegetables:* fresh fruit, dried fruit, vegetables.
4. *Breads and cereals:* whole-grain cereals, whole-grain breads, pastas.

It is not difficult to decide the number and quantities of foods to be selected from each group in order to have an adequate nutritional diet. The following pattern is recommended:

Milk	1 pint daily for adults (1½ pints for children)
Egg	1 egg (3 to 4 per week)
Protein	2 servings daily. May be extra milk, egg, cheese, meat alternate, legumes, nuts, or dishes made from these
Vegetables	1 medium-size potato daily
	1 average serving leafy, green or yellow vegetable daily
	1 average serving other vegetable daily
Fruits	1 average serving citrus fruit, tomato, or other rich source of vitamin C
	1 average serving other fruit (fresh, canned, or dried)
Butter	or fortified margarine, at least 2 tablespoons or 1 oz
Bread	and/or cereal—4 slices of whole-grain or enriched bread daily, or 3 slices whole-grain or enriched bread and 1 serving whole-grain cereal

The next step is to apply the previous information to meal planning for the day. The milk group may be divided among all three meals of the day taking into account the milk used in cooking. Proteins may also be divided among all three meals. Vitamins and minerals are usually portioned thus: for breakfast, a vitamin C fruit; for lunch and dinner, vegetables to be incorporated in both meals to supply the body amply, usually three servings daily. Breads and cereals may be divided as follows: cereal for breakfast, bread or toast for the other two meals.

In considering menu planning, the whole day should be kept in mind as a unit rather than just individual meals. Proteins, fats, and carbohydrates should be distributed throughout the day so that no meal will have a striking preponderance of one kind of fuel foodstuff. For example, a legume dish with macaroni and cheese concentrates the protein in one meal, potatoes with rice concentrate the carbohydrate, and fried potatoes and pie concentrate the fat. With the exception of a few staples such as bread, margarine, and milk, an effort should be made to avoid serving any food in the same form twice in the same day. Serving any food which gives character to a dish twice in the same meal, even in different forms, should be avoided. Example: tomato soup and tomato salad for the same meal. At each meal, contrasts should be sought between successive courses: a bland course followed by a more highly flavored course, and vice versa, to give a pleasing rhythm.

In each course attention should be paid to flavor, color, form, and texture. There are esthetic values in crisp crackers with soup, a green lettuce leaf on a salad plate, a red cherry on a rice pudding, a gelatin turned from a graceful mold, or a slice of lemon with a serving of greens. There are many other combinations with pleasing contrasts.

Since breakfast is an extremely important meal of the day, about one fourth to one third of the day's food should be eaten at breakfast. A hearty breakfast is an aid to eating less during the remainder of the day. The meal pattern should fit the individual needs of the members of the family. For example, the elderly will not need as much food as the growing adolescent.

Likes and dislikes should not dominate the choices made in the menu planning. Each member of the family should try to learn to like new foods.

Basic Menus

Breakfast

Fruit and/or fruit juice
Cereal with milk and/or bread with
  butter or margarine
Egg or other protein food
Beverage

Breakfast

Orange juice
Oatmeal with milk or cream
Toast with butter or margarine
Egg, hard or soft-cooked
Postum made with milk

Luncheon or Supper

Main dish or cream soup
Vegetable, raw or cooked, or fruit
Simple dessert or fruit
Bread with butter or margarine
Beverage

Luncheon or Supper

Macaroni and cheese or cream of
  green pea soup
Sliced tomato and lettuce
Peaches
Whole-wheat bread with butter or
  margarine
Milk

Dinner

High protein food
Potato or other starch food
Green or yellow vegetable
Salad or other cooked vegetable
Bread with butter or margarine
Fruit or dessert
Beverage

Dinner

Walnut loaf or soy cheese scallops
Medium potato, baked
Cooked carrots
Cabbage salad
Whole-wheat bread with butter or
  margarine
Custard
Milk

Effort should be made to remember to:

1. Eat a salad or raw vegetable every day if possible.
2. Eat a green-leafy or yellow vegetable every day.
3. Have a serving of citrus fruit, tomato, cantaloupe, strawberries, or raw cabbage every day.
4. Watch closely for "hidden calories" in food mixtures.
5. Keep enthusiasm high and the diet in sight.
6. Provide a variety from the Basic Four Food Groups.
7. Utilize seasonal foods.
8. Be adventurous in using new recipes.

Those concerned about a simple calorie guide for weight control may find the following 1000-calorie meal plan helpful.

1,000-Calorie Meal Plan

Breakfast

Fruit   2 servings
Egg   1
Cereal or toast   1 cup
*Milk, non-fat   1 cup
Butter or margarine   1 level teaspoon

Lunch or Supper

Protein foods   2 servings
Bread   1 slice
Vegetable Group 1   as desired
Vegetable Group 2   0
Fruit   1 serving
*Milk, non-fat   1 cup
Butter or margarine   0

*Buttermilk may be substituted for non-fat milk

Dinner

Protein foods   2 servings
Vegetable Group 1   as desired
Vegetable Group 2   1 serving
Bread list   ½ serving
Fruit   1 serving
*Milk, non-fat   1 cup
Butter or margarine   0

*Buttermilk may be substituted for non-fat milk

Helps for counting calories:

Breakfast	Calories	Dinner	Calories
1 Non-fat milk	80	2 Protein	150
1 Egg	75	½ Bread	34
2 Fruits (juices or		1 "B" vegetable	36
grapefruit)	80	"A" vegetable	Free
1 Bread	68	1 Fruit	40
1 Fat	45	1 Non-fat milk	80
Total	348	No fat	
		Total	340

Lunch	
2 Protein	150
1 Bread	68
A vegetable (broccoli)	Free
1 Fruit (orange)	40
1 Non-fat milk	80
Salad (tomato)	
No fat	
Total	338

Some Helpful Suggestions

1. Eating at regular times is important. Skipping meals should be avoided.

2. Celery sticks, tomatoes, broth, or a clear, hot beverage may be taken between meals if desired.

3. All necessary foods should be on hand. Meals for the entire day or for several days should be planned so the preparation is facilitated.

4. Fat should not be used in cooking unless it is part of the daily allowance.

5. If meat is used, it should be broiled, boiled, baked, or roasted. All visible fat should be removed before cooking.

6. Satisfaction is increased with leisurely eating.

7. Coffee, tea, or cola beverages are not recommended because they tend to be irritating or stimulating to the digestive and nervous systems. Decaffeinated coffee and herb teas may be substituted. Some herb teas are: orange, peppermint.

8. Small helpings or servings should be chosen. Seconds should be avoided.

Chapter 3

You Are What You Eat

About the turn of the century, the American population lived largely in rural areas. The people cultivated the soil, produced their own foodstuffs, and preserved their own food. There were no supermarkets in which to purchase supplies. Most of what people ate was made from their home-grown supplies. The foods contained natural nutrients. There was little so-called refinement of foods.

The author's mother comes from this generation, and memories are still vivid of the gardening, harvesting, and preserving from the labors of mother, father, and ten healthy children. Mother never had a course in nutrition, she never studied about diseases as they are known today, but she prepared balanced, tasty, and beautiful meals—full of natural nutrients. She has eaten her own cooking all her life; and, at eighty-eight, continues to bake and cook and is still well and happy.

As the children grew up, they lived a simple but complete and happy life. Everyone worked in the garden. Most of the early years were spent in northern Minnesota where it is hot in midsummer and cold in the winter, but home was comfortable. Family members shared in caring for the cows, horses, and chickens. In the summer season, 3,000 quarts of fruits and vegetables were canned. When fall harvest came along, roots were gathered (vegetables that grow underground) and carefully prepared for the cellar where they were placed in bins. There were enough potatoes, carrots, beets, rutabagas, parsnips, and cabbage to last through the winter; there was never a lack of enough tasty, wholesome food. There was no illness except perhaps the three-day measles "picked up" at school. As the cold winter set in, huge chunks of ice were cut from the frozen lakes, placed in the root cellar, and packed in clean sawdust to keep for the summer months. The ice provided refrigeration for milk and cream, and, of course, homemade ice cream for picnics and parties.

There were no refined foods; all foods were in their natural state. Those days are gone forever, for then came the advent of large-scale mechanized farming with modern methods of food preparation, changing the life-style and eating habits of the American people. Refined foods were produced in ever-increasing variety that brought changes in consistency and flavors with diminished nutritive values.

Today, what a contrast! Judging from the array of foods available, it might be assumed that the average American spends most of his time eating or thinking about where he will eat. Fast food restaurants or gourmet eating villas are close at hand. One may enter any super-market and choose from 12,000 or more items which are displayed in colorful arrangements. At work, vending machines or snack bars are near; at home, in his own kitchen, a variety of packages, cans, or boxes of food is available and requires only minutes to prepare.

The environment in which people eat directly affects the way they interpret and use nutritional information. Nutrient requirements are irrelevant if they cannot be translated into the mode of eating fol-lowed by those for whom the requirements were developed. As an example, lists of foods are checked to ensure the proper amounts of specific nutrients. Foods not familiar and easily obtainable at home and in the restaurants are seldom eaten. Rutabagas are a rich source of vitamin A, but how many people even recognize a rutabaga? How many fast food restaurants feature the rutabaga?

Working habits and disorganized home life often contribute the habit of skipping breakfast. For lunch, people run to the snack shop for a sandwich, and the day is half gone. Probably no well-balanced meal is eaten until evening, if then. At school, children are taught the Basic Four Food Groups; however, because of the varied ethnic groups, how many understand or can apply and follow the pattern? These practices illustrate how life-style affects the application of nutritional information.

The country is full of sick people today largely because of careless eating habits. It is high time that people return to the natural foods and eliminate the highly-refined sugar-coated "goodies."

The average American eats 17 percent or one fifth of his calories as sugar. According to statistics, enough sugar is consumed yearly to average over 100 pounds for every man, woman, and child in the United States. Excess sugar may pose problems because carbohy-drates require B vitamins for digestion. Sugar contains no B vitamins; consequently, in the utilization of other foods, there may be a short-age of these important vitamins. Therefore, sugar must steal them from other foods. Other problems resulting from eating too much sugar include dental caries, obesity, early heart attacks, infections, and increased body cholesterol.

How did this habit come about? Maybe a retrospective look will reveal the answer. In the early 1600s, sugar was known only as a curiosity. By the 1700s, sugar sold for one dollar per pound. In 1825, sugar sold for 25 cents per pound. At the time of the Revolutionary

War, the consumption of sugar per capita was 7½ pounds per year. Today the amount is over 100 pounds per person.

How much is 100 pounds of sugar per person? About 30 teaspoons each day. Most people are not aware of this fact because they are not spooning the sugar generously on foods. Rather, it is consumed "anonymously" in sweetened products. For example, the investment in soft drinks, which contain about 100 calories per eight-ounce bottle, is over five million dollars annually. Many people replace drinking water with sweetened carbonated drinks and juices.

The body needs carbohydrates for metabolism of fat, for protein-sparing action, and for furnishing the body with energy. The best sources of carbohydrates are natural sources such as fruits, grains, cereals, and a little from vegetables. Such sweeteners as sorghum, molasses, or sorbitol may be used. Artificial sweeteners have been used for a long time; however, they should not be used in excess. Honey is a sweetener, but it should be noted that it is a sugar and should be treated as a sugar. When the body receives too much carbohydrate, the excess is stored in the body as glycogen and fat.

Sometimes Americans are referred to as the "starving" Americans, not because they do not have food or cannot affort to buy it, but rather because much of the vast array of food at the shoppers' disposal is "junk food." There is an excess of highly refined foods such as breakfast cereals and pastries. Empty calories in abundance await the buyer. How about the billions of bottles of soda and liquor that are consumed daily? The abundance of misinformation, false advertising, claims for this and that, free for the listening and looking, are persuasive. Also, people are so busy keeping up with the pace of things that they do not have time for preparation of wholesome foods, so turn to something quick and easy. Furthermore, people do not take the time to eat regularly and choose wisely. Most other cultures in the world are not troubled with some of these common problems that Americans experience on a daily basis.

By using an abundance of sugar in the diet, people are cheating themselves of the important nutrients their bodies need, and are causing other deleterious effects. Sugar affects the membrane lining of the stomach and the intestines by extracting water from the tissues (holding hard candy in the mouth against the cheek soon demonstrates the need for water). Sugar also irritates by favoring fermentation in the stomach, thereby causing gas. One lump, or five grams, provides 20 calories. Excess calories that are not utilized result in obesity—a major health problem. Someone has said, "Everything I like is fattening," or "If it doesn't have calories, it isn't worth eating." These comments are classics, no? One out of three people in this country is overweight—fifty million people eating too much sugar!

* * *

This book is to help the reader make intelligent eating choices that will add quality years to life and provide a happier, healthier life during those years. Life-style and behavioral changes also are discussed to aid in making choices for the promotion of long-term weight management.

Chapter 4

Waistlines versus Lifelines

Magazines are full of articles pointing to new ways to lose weight, fast and easy ways, so the headlines say. Many gullible Americans will do most anything somebody suggests about dieting, and without evaluation. They go readily from one diet to another to lose those extra pounds. Bulges and rolls of fat not wanted and certainly not needed are the concern of more than 80 million Americans.

Who hasn't been on a diet of one kind or another many times, only to discover that as soon as it is over, the weight returns? A little porcelain plaque reads: "The pounds I lose come back in haste, to join their friends around my waist."

What then is wrong with most diets? For example, one well-known diet restricts carbohydrates to less than 40 grams per day, thus inducing a state of ketonuria (the excretion of ketone bodies in the urine). This diet is neither new nor revolutionary. The rationale advanced to justify it is, for the most part, without scientific merit, without concern for the "unlimited" intake of saturated fats and cholesterol-rich foods. Any grossly unbalanced diet is likely to induce some anorexia and weight reduction but can involve serious hazards.

Another diet that has swept the country calls for a "formula diet" that is taken until the desired weight is obtained. There is no change in life-style, and, as soon as the program is laid aside and old habits return, so does the weight. The liquid-protein diet is an example of another such diet. This one is apparently so dangerous that its sponsors advise that a physician monitor it because of possible adverse consequences. A fourth diet very popular today goes from specified fruits for a certain length of time to limited vegetables then to other specified foods for a definite number of days. Some of the foods in this diet are unavailable in many areas. This diet is dangerously incomplete and nutritionally unsound. Rice diets, grapefruit diets, fructose diets, and fasting diets may be dangerous and injurious to one's health if followed for a lengthy period. Any such diets should be followed under the advice and observation of a physician.

A person needing to lose weight should not consider fad diets, "miracle" foods, or magic pills that promise loss of many pounds in a relatively short period of time. A person planning to lose weight should keep in mind the importance of adequate nutrition, and should find out about the ideal types of "lifetime" foods the system needs if he wishes to operate at the peak of efficiency and to lose weight sensibly.

Correct eating does not mean staying on a boring, rigid diet that never varies. Correct eating is simply a matter of not overindulging, of eating a variety of nutritious, wholesome foods in controlled amounts. Correct eating is a matter of life-style and daily habits.

Taking weight off rapidly puts a heavy burden on the entire metabolic system, to say nothing of the dangers inherent in the so-called foolproof, fast diets, which are usually not nutritionally sound. Changing life's habits may not be easy for some people, but the effects and results are immensely rewarding. Carefully utilizing the simple program that follows in this chapter will build lasting success, and a happy and healthy personality—without unnecessary dangers. However, no plan is successful unless the person is determined about weight control.

The first step in a weight loss program is to set a realistic goal without fantasizing; that is, to be realistic as to the number of pounds to lose. The next step is to be cognizant of the time needed to reach this goal. Feeling better and looking better will be so rewarding that there will be little desire to revert to former habits.

The yo-yo syndrome of taking off ten pounds and putting on five should be avoided as the plague. The yo-yo game is a strain on the digestive system because the entire metabolic cycle is upset. The loss of two to three pounds per week is a safe goal. The yo-yo syndrome often accompanies crash diets because long-time habits have not been changed, and habits are the cause of the weight in the first place. The program recommended in this chapter is neither rigid nor to be followed for x number of days. There are no medications involved, nor do the amounts make for a starvation program, although at first the person may think he is starving if eating large amounts has previously been a habit. The person following the program should be determined to establish the new eating habits for the rest of his life—a new style for maximum living.

The noted American educator, Horace Mann, wrote, "Habit is a cable: we weave a thread of it every day and at last we cannot break it." Purpose, goal, and ambition should create the desire to change life-style eating patterns when necessary so a "cable" will be woven that cannot be broken.

The author's approach to weight control is habit-changing. If the new eating habits and exercise habits are maintained, weight will not only be lost but not regained. The reader should be ready to make some commitments, set a goal, and proceed with the task.

There are four important principles to follow.

Principle number one is *Do Not Eat Snacks* — absolutely *no* snacking at any time. This principle means no food to be eaten between meals: no cookies or doughnuts during rest breaks; no nibbling on potato chips or pastries; positively no refrigerator raids; no foods from candy, soft drink, or ice cream dispensers. Between-meal snacks are usually composed of highly refined, carbohydrate-loaded foods. Snack foods more often than not are very low in nutrients. By the time the meal hour rolls around, the habitual snacker is not hungry, so he nibbles. This person is not getting adequate nutrition. The snacker is also known to be a "binger" with little or no self-control. Sixty percent of the national population snacks.

The principle of no snacking is a behavioral change for some people. The snacking time should be replaced by a desirable activity other than eating. For some people, snacking is their biggest downfall and replacement is difficult. A help in making the change is to keep a record of all foods eaten during a 24-hour period. The information will aid in realizing what is currently being eaten as opposed to what should be eaten. The form below may be of assistance in evaluating amounts and kinds of foods eaten:

	Time	Kind and Amount of Food	Calories	Eating Place
Breakfast				
Lunch				
Dinner				

Using a notebook to keep a running record of the above is usually necessary. As the days, weeks, and months go by, dramatic changes in behavior will be evident.

Principle number two is *Eliminate Refined Foods*. Examples include rich desserts; candy; ice cream; highly processed grain products such as white bread, cookies, cakes, and doughnuts. Many packaged and bottled soft drinks that are high in sugar content, as well as alcoholic beverages, are full of "empty" calories. Two important reasons for eliminating such foods are: 1) refined and empty calorie foods tend to deplete the body's vitamin and mineral reserves, and 2) evidence indicates that refined sugar interferes with the body's ability to resist and fight disease.

Labels should be read carefully for contents. Hidden sugars are present in many cereals and canned foods including many brands of peanut butter and catsup. One soft drink alone may contain sugar from 15 feet of sugar cane. Or eight ounces of a soft drink, or a small candy bar, or a scoop of ice cream may have five or six teaspoons of sugar. One small slice of chocolate cake usually contains twelve teaspoons of sugar.

Fresh and dried fruit are excellent sources for the necessary carbohydrates the body needs. A helpful suggestion is to sweeten foods with dates, raisins, prunes, concentrated apple or orange juice. Refreshing substitutes for high-calorie desserts made from refined sugar are fresh fruits which are available in most places the year around. Honey is often used as a substitute for sugar; however, for equivalent quantities, honey has more calories than sugar.

Principle number three is *Decrease the Use of Visible and Invisible Fats*. Visible fats include table spreads, shortening, butter, salad dressings, cream cheese. Invisible fats are an integral part of such foods as milk, nuts, eggs.

There are two kinds of fats known as saturated and unsaturated. Saturated fats are those fats that are solid at room temperature, such as butter, lard, and some shortenings. Unsaturated fats are liquid at room temperature, such as corn, cottonseed, safflower, and soy oils. One exception is coconut oil which is high in saturated fatty acids despite the fact that it is a liquid.

By decreasing the use of visible and invisible fats, a remarkable decrease in total calories is obtained because fats contain over twice as many calories per gram as do proteins and carbohydrates.

Principle number four is *Eat a Nutritious Breakfast*. Starting the day with a nutritious breakfast is extremely important. Cooked cereals are better than the dry, packaged variety. If dry cereals are used, those containing unrefined grains plus a variety of fruits and nuts should be selected—for example, granola-type cereals. Puffed or popped varieties of the dry cereals are the least desirable. An adequate breakfast is important because calories taken early in the day are used to provide energy for work. Late, heavy dinners are often not digested easily and may be a contributing factor to ill health. High amounts of fat in the blood stream due to an excessive intake of calories not needed contribute to heart disease.

The four principles described above are vitally important. In summary, these simple ways to change life-long eating habits are:

1. Do not eat snacks.
2. Eliminate refined foods.
3. Decrease the use of visible and invisible fats.
4. Eat a nutritious breakfast.

Meals that include foods selected from the Basic Four Food Groups, described in Chapter 2, fulfill the above principles. All these foods are readily available. To insure variety and avoid dietary boredom, certain foods may be traded as substitutes for one another. These substitutions may be made from so-called exchange lists which provide variety, the spice of life.

What is an exchange list? This may be substitution or trade of one food for another. How does it work? An apple may be traded for an orange, half a banana for two apricots, a baked potato for a slice of bread, a teaspoon of mayonnaise for two tablespoons of sour cream. An exchange list has endless possibilities. The use of an exchange list brings not only variety, but interest and pleasure. Each day is an adventure.

An exchange list consists of groups of foods of comparable nutritional value that may be substituted for one another. The foods have been divided into seven groups or exchanges. To illustrate, vegetables are in one group, fats in another. Foods in any *one group* may be substituted or exchanged with any other foods in the *same group*.

In exchange lists, the words "exchange" and "serving" are used interchangeably. For example, 1 serving of cheese (1 oz.) = 1 protein exchange.

Protein Exchange List

Each serving provides: Protein, 7 gm; Fat, 5 gm; Calories, 73

Any kind of lean meat may be used. Eggs, most types of cheese, fish, poultry, and peanut butter may be used instead of meat for variety. A special listing is given for vegetarian meat substitutes.

Meat Should Be Weighed After It Is Cooked. A three-ounce portion of cooked meat is equal to four ounces of raw meat. Bones, skin, and extra fat should not be counted into the total weight since they are not eaten.

Weights are expressed as cooked meat or fish.

	Amount to Use
Meat and Poultry (medium fat) (beef, lamb, liver, chicken, etc.)	1 ounce
Egg (medium)	1
Beef Frankfurter (8–9 per pound)	1
Beef Franks, little (2 inches long)	2
Beef Sausages, link (15–16 per pound)	2
Fish	
Haddock, Halibut, Flounder, etc.	1 ounce
Herring (1 × 1½ × ½ inches)	1 piece
Salmon, Tuna	¼ cup
Fish Patties, frozen (omit ½ bread serving)	1 cake
Fish Sticks, frozen (omit ½ bread serving)	1½ sticks
Cheese	
Cheddar type	1 ounce
Cottage	¼ cup
Peanut Butter	2 tablespoons
(Limit to one serving a day unless the carbohydrate in peanut butter is allowed for in the meal plan.)	
Soy Beans	¼ cup

Meat substitutes: Worthington Foods, Battle Creek Foods*

Chic-Ketts (add ½ fat serving)	1 ounce (28 gm)
Cutlets, large size (add 1 fat serving)	½ piece (31 gm)

Fillets (omit ¼ fruit serving)	¾ stick (33 gm)
FriPats (omit ½ fruit serving)	½ FriPat (37 gm)
Fry Sticks (add ½ fat serving, omit ¼ fruit serving)	½ piece
GranBurger (add 1 fat serving, omit ¼ fruit serving)	½ ounce (14 gm) dehydrated

Luncheon Slices:

"Beef" Style, frozen (add ½ fat serving)	1 slice (28 gm)
"Chicken" style, frozen	1 slice (28 gm) or ¼ cup diced
Corned "Beef" Style (omit ½ fat serving)	3 slices (42 gm)
Madison Burger (add ¾ fat serving)	2 tablespoons & 2 teaspoons (29 gm)
Non-Meat Balls, canned	2 Non-Meat Balls (36 gm)
Prosage	⅜ inch slice (34.5 gm)
Protose	¼ inch slice (38 gm)
Salisbury Steak Style, frozen (omit ½ bread serving)	1 patty (57 gm)
Saucettes	2 links (34 gm)
Sandwich Spread	3 tablespoons
Smoked "Beef" Style (add ½ fat serving)	5 slices (35 gm)
Smoked "Turkey" Style	2 slices (38 gm)
Soymeat Diced Chicken Style (omit ½ fat serving)	1½ pieces (51 gm)
Stripples	5 slices (35 gm)
Stripple Zips (add ½ fat serving)	½ ounce (14 gm)
Veja-Links (omit 1 fat serving)	2 links (68 gm)
Vegetable Skallops (add 1 fat serving)	1½ pieces (43 gm)
Vegetable Steaks (add 1 fat serving)	2 pieces (40 gm)
Vegetarian Burger (add ½ fat serving)	2 tablespoons & 2 teaspoons (35 gm)

Meat substitutes: Loma Linda Foods*

Dinner Cuts (add 1 fat serving)	1 cut (44 gm)
Linketts	1
Proteena	¼ inch slice (37 gm)
Sandwich Spread (omit ½ fruit serving)	4 tablespoons
Vegebits (add 1 fat serving)	3 (44 gm)
Vegeburger (add 1 fat serving)	2 tablespoons (30 gm)
Vege-Chee	½ inch slice (70 gm)
Vege-Cuts (add 1 fat serving)	1 (43 gm)
Vegelona	¼ inch slice (47 gm)

---

*Worthington Foods, Inc., Worthington, OH 43085; Battle Creek Foods, Loma Linda Foods, 11503 Pierce St., Riverside, CA 92515.

Bread and Starch Exchange List

An example of the bread exchange is one serving of corn (⅓ cup) = 1 bread exchange.

Each serving provides: Protein, 2 gm; Carbohydrate, 15 gm; Calories, 68
Use whole-grain products often as allowable bread servings.

	Amount to Use
Bread	1 slice
Bagel	½ average
Biscuit, Roll (2-inch diameter)	1 average
Bread Crumbs	¼ cup
Bread Meal, Worthington (add 1 fruit serving)	1 tablespoon
Bread Sticks (8½ inches long)	2
Bread stuffing (omit 1 fat serving)	½ cup
Cinnamon Stick, Aunt Jemima (omit 1 fat serving)	2 sticks
Croutettes, Kellogg Co.	1 cup
Cornbread (1½ inch cube)	1
Corn Sticks, Aunt Jemima (omit 1 fat serving)	2 sticks
Frankfurter bun	1 small or ½ large
Hamburger bun	1 small or ½ large
Muffin (2-inch diameter)	1
Muffin, English	½ large
Popover (omit 1 fat serving)	1 average
Cornstarch	2 tablespoons
Flour	2½ tablespoons
Cereals, cooked	½ cup
Dry, flake	¾ cup
Dry, concentrated (All-Bran, Bran Buds)	⅓ cup
Granola	¼ cup
Shredded Wheat	1 biscuit
Pancake (4-inch diameter)	1 (¼ cup batter)
(omit ½ fat serving if not buttermilk pancake)	
Waffle, frozen (omit 1 fat serving)	1 pack (2)
(if homemade, each waffle, 5½-inch diameter, is 1½ bread servings)	
Hominy	⅓ cup
Rice, Grits, cooked	½ cup
Spaghetti, Noodles, Macaroni, cooked	½ cup
Chinese noodles (omit 1 fat serving)	½ cup
Crackers	
Graham (2½ inches square)	2
Oyster	20 or ½ cup
Saltines (2 inches square)	5
Soda (2½ inches square)	3
Round Thin (1½ inches)	6
Fritos (omit 2 fat servings)	⅔ cup
Matzo (6-inch diameter)	1
Matzo meal	3 tablespoons
Pizza (omit 1 fat serving)	⅛ of small pie
Poi	½ cup

Toast, melba (3½ × 1½ × ⅛ inches)	4 halves
Tortilla (6-inch diameter)	1
Wheat Germ	2 tablespoons
Vegetables	
Beans and peas, dried, cooked	½ cup
(lima, navy, split pea, cowpeas, pinto)	
Baked beans, no pork	¼ cup
Corn, whole kernel	⅓ cup
Corn, ear (5 × 1¾ inches)	1 ear
Parsnips	⅔ cup
Potatoes, white, baked or boiled (2-inch diameter)	1
Potatoes, white, mashed	½ cup
Potatoes, sweet or yams, no sugar added	¼ cup
Potato chips (2-inch diameter)	15 thin or 10 thick
(omit 2 fat servings)	
Potatoes, French-fried (½ × ½ × 2 inches)	⅔ cup
(omit 1 fat serving)	
Potatoes, shoestring (omit 2 fat servings)	6–8
Potatoes, Birds Eye frozen	
Potato Patties (omit 1 fat serving)	3 oz. (1 patty)
Potato Puffs (omit 2 fat servings)	⅓ package
Hash Browns	½ cup
Onion Rings, Birds Eye frozen (omit 2 fat servings)	2 oz. (½ small package or ⅓ large)
Popcorn, popped, unbuttered	1 cup
Cake, pound (2¾ × 3 × ⅝ inches)	1 slice
(omit 1 fat serving)	
Sponge cake, plain (1½ inch cube)	1
Jello, regular	⅓ cup
Ice Cream (omit 2 fat servings)	½ cup
Ice Milk (omit 1 fat serving)	½ cup
Sherbet	¼ cup
Vanilla wafers	5

Milk Exchange List

Each serving provides: Protein, 8 gm; Carbohydrate, 12 gm; Calories, 80

	Amount to Use
Non-Fat Fortified Milk	
Skim or non-fat milk	1 cup
Powdered (non-fat dry, before adding liquid)	⅓ cup
Canned, evaporated skim milk	½ cup
Buttermilk made from skim milk	1 cup
Yogurt made from skim milk (plain, unflavored)	1 cup
Low-Fat Fortified Milk	
1% fat, fortified milk* (omit ½ fat exchange)	1 cup
2% fat, fortified milk (omit 1 fat exchange)	1 cup
Yogurt made from 2% fortified milk (plain, unflavored) (omit 1 fat exchange)	1 cup

Whole milk (omit 2 fat exchanges)

Whole milk	1 cup
Canned, evaporated whole milk	½ cup
Buttermilk made from whole milk	1 cup
Yogurt made from whole milk (plain, unflavored)	1 cup

*1% fat milk may be prepared by mixing 2% fat milk with skim milk prepared from non-fat dried milk powder (according to package directions).

Fruit Exchange List

Each serving provides: Carbohydrates, 10 gm; Calories, 40

Fruit may be used fresh, canned or frozen, cooked or raw, as long as no sugar is added.

	Amount to Use
Apple (2-inch diameter)	1 small
Apple Juice	⅓ cup
Applesauce	½ cup
Apricot Nectar	⅓ cup
Apricots, fresh	2 medium
Apricots, dried	4 halves
Banana	½ small
Berries	
Blackberries	1 cup
Blueberries	⅔ cup
Raspberries	1 cup
Strawberries*	1 cup
Cantaloupe* (6-inch diameter)	¼
Cherries	10 large
Dates	2
Figs, fresh	2 large
Figs, dried	1 small
Fruit Cocktail	½ cup
Grapefruit*	½ small
Grapefruit Juice*	½ cup
Grapes	12
Grape Juice	¼ cup
Guava	1 small
Honeydew Melon (7-inch diameter)	⅛
Mandarin Oranges	¾ cup
Mango	½ small
Nectarine, fresh or unsweetened	1 medium
Orange*	1 small
Orange Juice*	½ cup
Papaya	⅓ medium
Peach	1 medium
Pear	1 small
Pineapple	½ cup
Pineapple Juice	⅓ cup
Plums	2 medium

Prunes, dried	2
Raisins	2 tablespoons
Tangerine*	1 large
Watermelon	1 cup

*These fruits are rich sources of vitamin C; one serving a day should be used.

Fats Exchange List

Each serving provides; Fat, 5 gm; Calories, 45

	Amount to Use
Avocado (4-inch diameter)	⅛
Butter or margarine	1 teaspoon
Chocolate, unsweetened, melted	2 teaspoons
Cream, light, sweet or sour	2 tablespoons
Cream, heavy	1 tablespoon
Half and Half	2 tablespoons
Cream Cheese	1 tablespoon
French Dressing	1 tablespoon
Gravies and Sauces	2 tablespoons
Mayonnaise	1 teaspoon
Nuts (if not specified below)	6 small
Almonds	8 whole
Brazil Nuts	2 whole
Cashews	5 whole
Hazelnuts or Filberts	6 whole
Pecans	6 halves
Pistachio	20 whole
Walnuts	5 halves
Oil	1 teaspoon
Olives	5 small

"A" Vegetables Exchange List

The generous use of many vegetables contributes to sound health and vitality when served either alone or in other foods such as casseroles, soups, or salads. If fat is added in the preparation, omit the equivalent of fat exchanges. The average amount of fat contained in a vegetable exchange that is cooked with animal or other fats is one fat exchange.

Asparagus	Cucumber	Peppers, Green or
Bamboo Shoots	Eggplant	Red*
Bean Spouts	Endive, Squash,	Radishes
Broccoli*	Zucchini	Rhubarb (without
Brussels Sprouts*	Escarole*	sugar)
Cabbage	Greens*	Sauerkraut
Cauliflower	Lettuce	String Beans, young
Celery	Mushrooms	Squash, Summer
Chicory*	Okra	Tomatoes**
	Parsley*	Water Cress*

*These vegetables have a high Vitamin A content; at least one serving a day should be used.
**Limit tomatoes to one average tomato or ½ cup tomato juice per meal.

"B" Vegetables Exchange List

Each serving provides: Protein, 2 gm; Carbohydrate, 7 gm; Calories, 36

All of these vegetables contain more carbohydrate than "A" vegetables. One half cup of the raw or cooked vegetable equals one serving. Raw, cooked, canned, or frozen vegetables may be used.

Artichokes	Onions	Rutabagas
Beets	Peas, Green	Squash, Winter*
Carrots*	Pumpkin	Turnips
Mixed Vegetables		

In addition, vegetables frozen in butter sauce have 1 fat serving per ½ cup.
*These vegetables have a high vitamin A content; at least one serving a day should be used.

Free Foods

At each meal as many servings of the following free foods as one desires may be taken since they contain negligible calories.

Clear Bouillon, fat free
Clear Broth, fat free
Cocoa Powder, unsweetened
Cranberries, unsweetened
Dietetic Jellies and Jams, sugar-free
D'Zerta brand Gelatins
Gelatin, unsweetened
Herbs, Spices, Seasonings except:
   Soy Sauce (limit to 1 tablespoon)
   Worcestershire Sauce (limit to 1 tablespoon)
Kaffir Tea
Lemon
Mint
Pickles, sour
Pickles, unsweetened dill
Pimento
Postum
Rennet Tablets
Saccharin and other non-caloric sweeteners
Salad Dressings, non-caloric or very low-caloric
Soft Drinks, sugar-free
Vinegar
V-8 Cocktail Vegetable Juice (limit to ½ cup)
Water
Yogurt, skimmed, unflavored (limit to 2 tablespoons per day)

The foods in each exchange list are familiar, everyday foods. Familiarity with the exchange lists will reveal that some foods are not mentioned. The following foods should be avoided in the diet plan: sugar, candy, honey, jam, jelly, cookies, syrup, condensed milk, chewing gum, soft drinks, pies, cakes, and ice cream. Also, one should use a minimum of table salt, preferably substituting other seasonings.

Following are suggested daily meal plans including various caloric levels. Selections of foods should be based on the level that best provides the energy needed.

Daily Meal Plans: Daily Exchanges

To use the meal plan for 800 calories, the exchanges are divided into three meals. From the *"A" Vegetables Exchange List,* use as desired. From the *"B" Vegetables Exchange List,* 1 vegetable is chosen. From the *Bread and Starch Exchange List,* 2½ exchanges are chosen. From the *Protein Exchange List,* 5 exchanges are chosen. From the *Milk Exchange List,* 1 non-fat milk is chosen. From the *Fruit Exchange List,* 3 fruit exchanges are chosen. From the *Fats Exchange List,* 1 fat exchange is chosen.

By following the guidelines in this and other chapters in this book one may set up a life-long regime that will be successful. The necessary information to insure longer living is contained in this volume. Waistlines and lifelines are the reader's challenge and choice.

One more important component that must be included to control waistlines is exercise. Exercise may be done by walking for one half hour every day. Other exercises may be preferred; however, there should be a definite exercise program, followed every day.

Calories		800	1000	1200	1500	1800	2000	2200	2500	3000	Page
"A" Veg. Exchange		AD	AD	AD	AD	AD	AD	AD	AD	AD	36
"B" Veg.	"	1	1	1	1	1	1	1	1	1	37
Bread	"	2½	3	4½	5½	7½	9½	10½	12	13½	33
Protein	"	5	6	6	6	7	8	8	8	10	31
Milk	"	1nf	1nf	1nf	2nf	2nf	2nf	4nf	4nf	5nf	34
Fruit	"	3	4	4	4	4	3	4	5	6	35
Fat	"	1	2	4	7	9	9	9	11	14	36

AD—as desired
nf—non-fat

Chapter 5

Start Your Day with an Adequate Breakfast

By the happiest of coincidences, life's fundamental necessity is also one of life's supreme pleasures—*Food*. Questions that may be asked include: are the right foods being eaten, in the right amounts, at the right time, in order to supply the required nutrients to meet the body's daily needs? Eating too little makes the body draw from its reserve resources. Eating too much causes obesity.

The Senate Select Committee on Nutrition and Human Needs published a report entitled, "Dietary Goals for the United States." This report called for major changes in the average American diet. Among the report's suggestions were an increase of fruits and vegetables, a decrease in the amount of cholesterol, a decrease in the amount of fats, and a decrease in the amount of sugar. These suggestions would indicate that the average American is not the best-fed person in the world. In fact, other studies indicate that Americans are among the poorest-fed people in the world. This condition is not caused by a lack of nutritious food, nor does it indicate that the economy is such that people cannot afford nutritious food. The real reasons are that poor choices are made from the wide selection available, and there is an oversupply of rich and refined foods.

Many diet histories reveal that people tend to eat little or no fruits and vegetables, too many sweets, pastries, and starches; they drink generously of carbonated beverages; and they tend to snack throughout the day, seldom eating a balanced nutritious meal. Little thought and effort go into eating the proper foods, in the proper amounts, to supply the daily nutrients that are vital to maintaining optimal health.

The day should start with a nutritious breakfast. This is the most important meal of the day. Every body cell has "rested," and, after a fast with a night's rest, the cells are calling for energy. This energy is supplied by eating a wholesome, nutritious breakfast that will supply the power to meet the day's demands. The lack of a nutritious breakfast affects the disposition. If the body is deprived of its energy source, irritability and impatience result. But a satisfactory breakfast contributes to well-being and an appearance of freshness and vigor. No meal offers more opportunity and delight than breakfast, and a brunch presents a joyously relaxed occasion for entertaining.

In conducting weight management clinics, the participation of each member of the class is invited by asking pertinent questions. Inquiries about breakfast bring interesting responses and many excuses for not eating breakfast. Some say that they are not hungry. The main reason that people are not hungry is because they usually overeat at a late hour the night before. Others say there is not adequate time. But everyone has 24 hours to spend as he pleases. He must eat, sleep, work, play, and relax. One usually finds time to do the things he really wants to do.

One should take time for an adequate breakfast, plan for it the night before so that rushing in the morning is not necessary. Breakfast is a meal of togetherness when the family sets the pace and tone for the day.

Some people just don't like to eat early in the morning. Some folk are watching their weight so choose breakfast as an easy meal to skip. Surveys show that half or less adults eat an adequate breakfast. Still more tragic is the fact that about 80 percent of children eat an inadequate breakfast or skip it altogether. Studies done in Iowa, Connecticut, and New Jersey indicate that breakfasts are the poorest meal of the day.

What are some of the results when little or no breakfast becomes a way of life? Usually by 10 a.m. there is a big letdown, and coffee, a doughnut, or maybe a candy bar is eaten for energy. This type of eating is high in carbohydrates, low in protein, low in vitamins and minerals. Therefore, the body is forced to call on its reserves. This practice may cause nervousness, irritability, and other undesirable behavior.

Breakfast often provides much of the daily requirement for calcium found in milk. When there is deficiency, the body is forced to take calcium from the bones and teeth. Usually the person is deficient in total daily nutritional intake. The foods eaten for breakfast supply nutrients that are not usually obtained in other meals.

For the individual who cannot use regular milk, a specially formulated, easily digestible product, LactAid, is available. LactAid is 70 percent lactose reduced, low-fat milk. LactAid has a natural enzyme added to reduce milk lactose into a simpler, more digestible form.

There are many different combinations of food which make a tasty and well-balanced breakfast. Following are some basic principles to use as a guide in planning a menu at different cost levels.

1. A well-balanced breakfast menu should contain one fourth to one third of the total day's needs of all nutrients.

2. The choice of food should complement the rest of the meals for the day, with balance in flavor and nourishment.

3. The menu should be one that can be prepared in the time allotted.

4. The menu should please the tastes of the family: different grains for breads and cereals, a diversified arrangement of fruits.

Whole-grain cereals are strongly recommended. Refined cereals lose much of their nutritional values, and the cost is increased. For example, 13 of the nutrients in wheat are decreased as follows in the refining process:

Percent		Percent	
86	Vitamin B_1 Thiamine	50	Calcium
70	Vitamin B_2 Riboflavin	78	Phosphorus
86	Niacin	75	Copper
60	Vitamin B_6	72	Magnesium
70	Folic Acid	71	Manganese
54	Pantothenic Acid	84	Iron
90	Biotin		

By the "enriching" process, B_1, B_2, niacin, and iron may be added, but in what amounts—and what about other nutrients? These may not be obtained from other foods in the day's meals. Whole grains may be compared to "diamonds"—they are full of important elements that should not be removed by refining.

The reader is urged to avoid "empty" calories, refined foods, excessive fats, sugar, syrups, and candies, and to eat foods containing vitamins, minerals, and protein from natural sources.

Cereals may be enhanced by the addition of one or more of the following:

1. Grated apple
2. Sliced fresh peaches
3. Grated coconut
4. Wheat germ
5. Ground nuts
6. Fresh berries
7. Brewer's yeast
8. Ripened persimmon
9. Chopped dates or figs
10. Sliced bananas
11. Raisins

An artistic touch can make the humblest object into a masterpiece of beauty. Awareness of beauty in food characterizes the food artist who makes every meal a work of art, inviting to see and to eat.

A few low-calorie ideas for breakfast may be helpful.

Low-Calorie Breakfast Menus

1. Tomato juice
   Scrambled egg on toast
   Milk or hot cocoa

2. Chilled V-8 juice
   Toasted cheese sandwich
   Milk

3. Whole-grain cereal
Hard-boiled egg
Milk
Orange

4. Soy waffle
Applesauce and peanut
butter
Margarine
Milk

5. Whole-wheat toast with
Applesauce and cottage
cheese
Milk

6. Open-faced sandwich
Sliced tomatoes and cheese
Milk

7. Poached egg on whole-wheat
toast
Orange
Milk

8. Granola Bars
Fresh fruit
Milk

9. Bran muffin
Fresh fruit
Milk
Cottage cheese

10. Cheese omelet
Grapefruit half
Milk
Whole-wheat toast

The busy executive who might have unexpected demands should not omit breakfast, but rather have something at hand that can be obtained readily.

1. A whole-grain muffin and a glass of milk
2. A granola bar and a glass of milk
3. A fruit and nut cookie and a glass of milk
4. A sandwich made the night before
5. A fruit yogurt and wheat crackers
6. A bag of seeds or nuts
7. Alfa-Mint tea or a fruit juice to replace coffee

Any one or a combination of the foods listed is much better than omitting the breakfast meal. Nuts and seeds are a high-protein mini-meal. Nuts and seeds also contain fat, which means calories. Some nuts contain less fat than others. Nutritional winners are peanuts and almonds; sunflower, pumpkin, and sesame seeds. These are all sources of calories, containing extraordinary amounts of protein, fiber, polyunsaturated fat (except sesame seeds), and almost the entire chart of vitamins and minerals.

Sugar Content, Breakfast Cereals

Many cold breakfast cereals contain the sugars sucrose and glucose. This chart shows percentages of sucrose and glucose in commercial breakfast cereals.

Cereal Product	Sucrose Content %	Glucose Content %	Cereal Product	Sucrose Content %	Glucose Content %
Shredded Wheat	1.0	0.2	40% Bran Flakes		
Shredded Wheat			(Kellogg)	10.2	2.1
(spoon)	1.3	0.3	Granola........	16.6	0.6
Cheerios	2.2	0.5	100% Bran	18.4	0.8
Puffed Rice	2.4	0.4	All Bran........	29.0	1.5

Cereal Product	Sucrose Content %	Glucose Content %	Cereal Product	Sucrose Content %	Glucose Content %
Uncle Sam Cereal	2.4	1.2	Granola (with almonds and filberts)	21.4	1.2
Wheat Chex	2.5	0.9	Fortified Oat Flakes	22.2	1.2
Grape Nut Flakes	3.3	0.6	Heartland	23.1	3.2
Puffed Wheat	3.5	0.7	Super Sugar Chex	24.5	0.8
Alpen	3.8	4.7	Sugar Frosted Flakes	29.0	1.8
Post Toasties	4.1	1.7	Bran Buds	30.2	2.1
Product 19	4.1	1.7	Sugar Sparkled Corn Flakes	32.2	1.8
Corn Total	4.4	1.4	Frosted Mini Wheats	33.6	0.4
Special K	4.4	6.4	Sugar Pops	37.8	2.9
Wheaties	4.7	4.2	Alpha Bits	40.3	0.6
Corn Flakes (Kroger)	5.1	1.5	Sir Grapefellow	40.7	3.1
Peanut Butter	5.2	1.1	Super Sugar Crisp	40.7	4.5
Grape Nuts	6.6	1.1	Cocoa Puffs	43.0	3.5
Corn Flakes (Food Club)	7.0	2.1	Cap'N Crunch	43.3	0.8
Crispy Rice	7.3	1.5	Crunch Berries	43.4	1.0
Corn Chex	7.5	0.9	Kaboom	43.8	3.0
Corn Flakes (Kellogg)	7.8	6.4	Frankenberry	44.0	2.6
Total	8.1	1.3	Frosted Flakes	44.0	2.9
Rice Chex	8.5	1.8	Count Chocula	44.2	3.7
Crisp Rice	8.8	2.1	Orange Quangaroos	44.7	0.6
Raisin Bran (Skinner)	9.6	9.3	Quisp	44.9	0.6
Concentrate	9.9	2.4	Boo Berry	45.7	2.3
Rice Crispies (Kellogg)	10.0	2.9	Vanilly Crunch	45.8	0.7
Raisin Bran (Kellogg)	10.6	14.1	Baron Von Redberry	45.8	1.5
Heartland (with raisins)	13.5	5.6	Cocoa Krispies	45.9	0.8
Buck Wheat	13.6	1.5	Trix	46.6	4.1
Life	14.5	2.5	Froot Loops	47.4	0.5
Granola (with dates)	14.5	3.2	Honeycomb	48.8	2.8
Granola (with raisins)	14.5	3.8	Pink Panther	49.2	1.3
Sugar Frosted Corn Flakes	15.6	1.8	Cinnamon Crunch	50.3	3.2
40% Bran Flakes (Post)	15.8	3.0	Lucky Charms	50.4	7.6
Team	15.9	1.1	Cocoa Pebbles	53.5	0.6
Brown Sugar Cinnamon Frosted Mini Wheat	16.0	0.3	Apple Jacks	55.0	0.5
			Fruity Pebbles	55.1	1.1
			King Vitamin	53.5	3.1
			Sugar Smacks	61.3	2.4
			Super Orange Crisp	68.0	2.8

Journal of Dentistry for Children, Sept.–Oct., 1974

Almonds contain 19 percent protein, B vitamins, vitamin E, magnesium (for a healthy heart), iron, and fiber. While almonds are 50 percent fat, these fats are mostly unsaturated and rich in linolenic acid, a component of fat associated with lower blood pressure.

From *Executive Fitness Newsletter,* March, 1984: pumpkin seeds contain an amazing 20 percent protein; sunflower seeds have 24 percent protein and are high in potassium and low in sodium, a combination of the two minerals that experts believe may lead to lower blood pressure. Sesame seeds are high in protein but also high in saturated fats. However, they are providers of a substance called sesamal, an antioxidant that some researchers believe can protect against cancer.

Protein and Fat Content of Nuts

Amount: 100 gm. or 3 oz. weight. *Volume:* approx. ½ cup plus 1–2 Tablespoons.

	Protein	Fat	Calories
Almonds	18.6	54.2	598
Brazil nuts	14.3	66.9	645
Cashews	17.2	45.7	561
Coconut (dried, unsweetened. 1 cup plus 4 teaspoons)	7.2	64.9	662
Peanuts	26.0	47.5	564
Pecans	9.2	71.2	687
Filberts (Hazel Nuts)	12.6	62.4	634
Sesame Seeds (whole)	18.6	49.1	563
Sunflower Seeds	24.0	47.3	560
Walnuts	14.8	64.0	651

Noteworthy: highest fat content, *pecans;* lowest fat content, *cashews.*

Information taken from Agriculture Handbook No. 8, Agricultural Research Service, U.S. Dept. of Agriculture.

Caution: Raw cashew nuts may be dirty and should be washed before using. Before using them uncooked, they should be washed and sterilized by baking on a cooking sheet at 200° F. for 1½ to 2 hours.

Chapter 6

Exercise for Total Health

Exercise, why bother? Lack of exercise affects the working of the body in four areas: strength of muscles, flexibility of joints, efficiency of the heart and lungs, and circulation of blood.

The body needs exercise just as it needs food. Exercise increases the circulation of the blood, causes deep breathing, and affects body tone. Activity not only helps in controlling weight, but it improves one's outlook on life and removes boredom and depression. Everyone should exercise at a pace that is comfortable and acceptable. Unlike a machine, the body wears out faster when it is idle than when it is used.

In maintaining adequate fitness, however, one does not need to make exercise into unpleasant, hard work. Each person should realize his limitations. Exercise can be a simple activity. Walking is a simple pleasure, but it has been overshadowed by such glamorous sports as tennis, skiing, swimming, and a host of others. Some people have joined expensive spa programs in order to reassert control over their lives and energies, to recharge their batteries, to improve their health. Yet, all one has to do is to stretch the legs and start walking. Walking is one of the best exercises for everyone in general. With few exceptions, anyone can walk. One should choose the best time, but walk for exercise, for fun, for improved living. "Exercising may start at any age and the body will respond," says Hulda Crooks of Loma Linda University, who is a renowned mountain climber at age 87.

Walking in the early morning stimulates efficiency of the body in delivering oxygen to the cells. It tones the muscles and joints and clears the mind for starting the day. Seeing the bright sunrise, listening to the birds, watching a squirrel climb a tree, seeing a deer jump out of the brush, or watching a jackrabbit bounce across the path—all of these attractions along the way are fun.

Just before retiring at night, some people enjoy riding an exercycle for 30 minutes. Then, when bedtime arrives, the body is relaxed, tired, and ready for a night's rest.

Time for exercise should be planned—made a top priority of daily living, one that supercedes work, fun, or any other activity that might appear more enticing. Thinking there is not enough time for exercising is just a "cop-out." A walk may be enjoyed by simply getting up 30 minutes earlier than usual. Everyone has 24 hours every day to use as he wishes: work, cook, eat, clean, tend to the children, keep the home going. To have time for each day's program requires organization and planning, including time for appropriate exercise and personal care. Each family member is important to himself and to the family. This importance and pleasure increase when health is "tops," disposition is "sweet," and the day's activities are organized to accomplish all that needs to be done. Exercise should not be considered as taking too much time. The company of a friend or family member may add to the pleasure of the exercise—someone that has similar interests and needs, so that sight of the ultimate goal is not lost. Varying routes when walking may add interest.

Increased health and happiness come from observing Nature's offerings: sunshine, fresh air, nutritious foods. Today people are plagued with polluted air, physical inactivity, lack of sleep, tension, indulgence of appetite, and frequently the use of drugs, including alcohol and tobacco.

A return to the simple life contributes to "life abundant." People tend to be slaves of their environment, jobs, ambitions. Real determination and a strong will are necessary if the pattern of behavior is to be improved. Some people are afraid to change, while others pay hundreds and thousands of dollars to go to a conditioning center to have their patterns of behavior altered. Actually, a change of life-style can begin right at home. First of all, the importance of adhering to health principles must be recognized. Maybe fewer dollars will be earned, but recreation is important instead of only entertainment. Time spent on frivolous social fraternizations may be devoted to increased time with the family, learning to enjoy one another. Life is valuable, meaningful, precious. To neglect the body is expensive.

Exercising applies to all daily activities. One should think of the routine that is followed daily and make a list of all the shortcuts that are taken. Then study the routine a bit and make a list of activities that could be incorporated on a regular basis. These suggestions might apply:

1. Take stairs when possible in place of the elevators.
2. Walk when possible instead of driving.
3. Indulge in bicycling, swimming, hiking, bowling, croquet.
4. Research recreational resources.
5. Create opportunities to exert.
6. At parties, don't just sit, circulate.
7. Avoid conveniences when possible.
8. Look for an active friend to join in the activities.

By taking the easy path, one could be sacrificing health.

Most doctors agree that the agent responsible for improving mental health, as one becomes physically fit, is the hormone, noradrenaline. Noradrenaline is believed to act as a stimulant, increasing alertness, reducing fatigue, and assisting in concentration. Balanced by proper exercise, noradrenaline can tone up the body and produce glow and mental tone that are associated with total health.

Muscles get smaller when not adequately exercised. Apart from affecting physical strength, strong muscles are necessary to pump sufficient blood to the heart. The heart is a miracle muscle and requires exercise to function efficiently. The heart will become smaller when the stimulation of physical activity is neglected. The circulation of the blood can be affected by the lack of exercise. When tiny vessels of the circulatory system close up, increasing the risk of a heart attack or a stroke, the lack of exercise may be a contributing cause.

Athletes need to train for many hours to achieve performance that wins in competition. Becoming physically fit means improving the condition of the body so the daily demands may be met comfortably.

Exercise is doubly important to the person who is attempting to lose weight. The task of burning extra calories is a major consideration. David Levitsky, Ph.D., Cornell University, in an article published in *Tufts University Diet and Nutrition Letter*, Vol. 1, No. 12, Feb., 1984, suggests that "The timing of exercise in relation to eating and not just exercise alone, may be important to individuals trying to control their weight." He also says that if one engages in exercise an hour or so after eating, he may burn off more calories than if he exercises on an empty stomach, and exercise performed a day after the overindulgence may cause the body to "waste" calories, so that one does not gain as much weight as one would expect. This observation would indicate that when one exercises for weight control, both what one does and when one does it are important.

There are many exercises to be considered. The author only wishes the reader to become inspired enough to become involved, choose what fits him best, and determine to exercise on a regular basis at a given time. The following simple routine may be only an example of exercises to be followed on a regular basis:

Hip and Thigh Exercises

I. *Lying with back on the floor*
1. Bicycle in the air with both legs, alternating to left and right and back to the middle (use as warm-up).
2. Left leg bent, right leg straight up in the air, turn right leg inward and outward as descending leg back down to floor; alternate with other leg.
3. With both legs straight on the floor, lift right leg up with knee bent, straighten out into the air and cross leg over left leg, then bring back and down to starting position and repeat with other leg to opposite side.

II. *Sitting on the floor*
1. "Walk" forward and backward on buttocks until the seat feels comfortably warm.
2. Roll over the hips to the left, straighten out right leg while lifting it up off the floor, roll back and do the same to other side.
3. Spread legs slightly, lift up right leg and bring it up diagonally toward the left, bring it back down again. Repeat with other leg.

III. *Sidelying*
1. Lift top leg up toward ceiling, bottom leg is bent, knee of top leg is straight, and toes are pointing forward; turn leg inward and outward coming down slowly while turning. Repeat a few times, then turn to other side.
2. Lift up top leg in same manner as high as possible, then touch down with toes down in front, lift leg up again and touch down with heel behind. Do a few times, then change to other side.
3. Start making small circles with top leg, slowly increase them in size, reduce them again and rest. Try to build up to at least 3–5 circles each time. Turn over and do same thing with the other side.

IV. *Standing* (Hold on to back of chair or similar object for stability.)
1. Bend right knee toward chest, straighten knee out slowly, then bring it down slowly. Repeat with left leg.
2. Make small circles with one leg mainly toward the side (knee is straight, foot pulled up). Increase the circles in size as much as possible. Slowly decrease again and stop. Alternate with other leg.
3. Hold on to chair and start with "little" kneebends, eventually try to get down as far as possible. When coming up, do not pull with the hands, but push the weight with the legs.

The following references may be helpful to consult when planning an exercise program:

1. *Exercise: The Why and the How,* by Paul Vodak, The Bull Publishing Company, P. O. Box 208, Palo Alto, California 94302.
2. *Feel Younger, Live Longer,* by Jack Tresidder, Rand McNally and Company, New York, Chicago, San Francisco.
3. *Diet and Exercise Guide,* by Mary Milo, Beauty Editor and Family Circle Food Staff, The Family Circle, Inc., a Subsidiary of the New York Times Media Company, Inc.

Chapter 7

Weigh to Stay

A language specialist claims that the five sweetest phrases in the English language are: "I love you," "Dinner is served," "All is forgiven," "Sleep until noon," "Keep the change," and those who have gained the victory over weight have added this one, "You've lost weight."

To follow a plan in which life-styles are changed means dedication to total health. By now the reader is aware that there are elements that are vital to change. So far this volume has been concerned with only two components vital for total health. One component is diet and another is exercise. At no time is a specific diet suggested. Rather, a plan is suggested that may be adapted to meet individual needs. The exchange system lists have wide acceptance in food selection, and are easy to understand and follow. These lists provide latitude for likes and dislikes. Food exchanges are listed in Chapter 4.

An exercise program should receive daily participation. Too many calories taken in and too few expended spell extra pounds. Some people don't count calories, and they have a "figure" to prove it. "Eat what you should and not what you could." This slogan is worth thinking about. Too many people do just the opposite and apologize for their indulgence while seemingly doing negligible exercising. Exercise should become a habit. Some exercises make the figure firm, others help slim down the figure.

The guidelines discussed in this chapter are to help the reader to manage weight and enjoy health. Meal patterns similar to those given for weight reduction should become a long-term practice. After four weeks, some people may need to continue the weight-loss program; if so, the program undertaken should be continued until the goal is achieved. When the goal is achieved, the exchange list may be consulted to choose which kinds and amounts of foods to increase or decrease in order to maintain the desired weight.

To prevent overweight involves a lifetime of intelligent habits. Here are a few tips on weight control:

1. Use the daily Basic Four Food Groups for the meals—no crash diets.
2. Satisfy all nutrient needs with a wide variety of different foods.
3. Eat at regular hours—not more than three meals per day.
4. Start each day with a nutritious breakfast—skippers tend to snack.
5. Refuse between-meal snacks.
6. Eat light suppers—two meals per day may be sufficient for some people.
7. Eat unrefined foods—these have less empty calories.
8. Use fruits for dessert—a fruit in place of a piece of pie.
9. Eat less fat.
10. Watch potluck and cafeteria traps that may encourage overeating.
11. Chew food thoroughly, eat slowly, avoid second helpings.
12. Have regular times for exercise. Push away from the table at the right time. Remember the "battle of the bulge" can't be won by diet alone.
13. Remember to think thin, stay slim, never lose sight of the goal. (Enjoy the reward of a new garment when the weight goal is achieved.)

Avoid the "yo-yo syndrome"—losing and gaining on a regular basis is not conducive to maintaining and enjoying ultimate health.

Many working people have jobs that determine the time and place for meals. The evening meal may be the only time a family is together. Therefore, the evening meal may be the heartiest meal of the day. In such cases, one would be well advised to have an exercise program in the evening. Such a program has its own rewards. The metabolic processes speed up, the calories are burned more readily, and the family has the opportunity to enjoy togetherness.

For the retired person the life-style may be simpler. Careful consideration should be given to decreasing foods in the evening meal and increasing foods for breakfast. Many retirees choose to eat two meals, starting near 9:30 a.m. or so for breakfast, lunch at 2:00 p.m., and perhaps only fruit at night. Each one must determine what is best in meeting his individual needs.

Motivation, as psychiatrists will often say, is difficult to assess. It is particularly difficult to trace in the murky sea of dieting and exercising. Some enjoy the excitement of the battle, but fail to note the implications or the consequences. Some admire the virtues of motivation in other people and at other times, but fail to comprehend its current potentialities. Courage, determination, and willpower are needed to battle one's eating habits and control weight. The differences in motivation between one person and another, the reasons that one achieves goals and another does not, are indeed complex. There is a mysterious relationship between the mind and the body; they react upon each other. Therefore, to keep the body in a healthy condition, all parts of the living machinery must act harmoniously. To neglect the body is to neglect the mind.

A review of a few facts about the human body may be of interest. The brain weighs a little over three pounds. The nerves are all connected to it, directly or by the spinal cord. These nerves with all their branches number in the millions. The amount of blood in an adult averages 30 pounds, or one fifth of the body weight. The heart is about six inches long and four inches across, and beats about 70 times a minute, 4,200 times an hour, 100,800 times a day, 36,792,000 times a year; at each beat two and a half ounces of blood are pumped through it—the equivalent of 175 ounces a minute, 656 pounds an hour, for a total of 7¾ tons a day. All the blood in the body passes through the heart in three minutes.

The lungs contain about one gallon of air when normally filled. A person breathes on the average 1,200 times an hour, inhaling about 24,000 gallons of air a day. The body has 206 bones. Collectively, there are over 600 different muscles in the human body. The digestive tract is about 30 feet long. The skin is made up of two layers and varies from one fourth to one eighth of an inch in thickness. Each square inch of skin has about 35,000 pores.

Man is marvelously made. Whoever is curious and eager to investigate the wonderful body and mind does not have to search the world, but only to examine himself.

Goal-setting is extremely important. One needs to be realistic and keep the goal always in mind. No one can afford extra calories on an ongoing basis. Once life-styles have been changed and the habits are established, carelessness should not be allowed to interfere with the original goals and objectives.

Chapter 8

You Are in Charge

Self-concept is a subjective constellation of past and present experiences, memories, physical perceptions, and all that goes into what is called "a person." A person feels either positive about "himself" or negative. A positive self-concept is certainly important. One should learn to concentrate on self-worth and never underestimate oneself.

Perhaps the major factor related to self-worth is identity—"who am I, why am I here, where am I going?" In order to live the life that counts, the spiritual, mental, and physical needs must be met.

The everyday occurrences, the mundane activities that are met each day, take on a new meaning when the mental attitude is positive. Positive thinking is very important. The pessimist provides an illustration in point. Two friends were visiting on a beautiful, clear day, following several days of snow, wind, and bitter cold. One remarked how nice the weather was and how much she was enjoying it. The answer was, "Well, it won't last long. It will probably rain before the day is over and be all dark again. You can't trust the weather any more," and on and on, in this same vein. Needless to say this person's mind was made up, but the companion was a positive thinker who went right on enjoying Mother Nature. How much better to think positively, to think or read something uplifting every day, something that will add a plus to a person's mental store of knowledge! Positive thinking is a part of healthful living. To have a positive outlook on life is important in feeling well, in accomplishing worthwhile goals.

Qualification for success is acquired through habit. Man is a bundle of habits; men form habits, and habits form futures. If one does not deliberately form worthwhile habits, then he will unconsciously form undesirable ones. Each person is the kind of person he is because he formed the habit of being that kind of a person, and the only way he can change for the better is through changing his habits.

Success is a habit. Failure is also a habit. Man chooses his own pattern of thought. He makes his own blueprints of his future. Man creates his own success but he also creates his own failures. Success is not an accident; the key is to acquire the right habits.

Thinking is a function of the mind. Thinking is a process, not some physical object you can see. Mind is a process for digesting experience. Man's greatest asset is his mind, for the mind is the door to the heart and the soul. The human creature has enormous capacity to set himself straight if he is given opportunity to think things out for himself. People get what they want in this world only after they have formed a clear picture of what they want.

A mysterious relationship exists between the mind and the body. They react upon each other. Therefore, to keep the body in a healthy condition, all parts of the living machinery must act harmoniously. To neglect the body is to neglect the mind. How may choices be made to insure the best possible care of the body? Following are some simple suggestions to help:

The body needs *Exercise* of some type every day. The reader might wish to refer to Chapter 6 for more details and direction in exercise.

A vital need is to drink plenty of pure, fresh *Water* to aid in the digestion of food and in the elimination of waste products. One should drink six to eight glasses of water during the day. Large quantities of liquid should be avoided at meals because they dilute the digestive juices and weaken the digestive processes.

Rest is another vital ingredient that is very important to health. Planning the day's program should include adequate time for sleep and rest. Eight hours a day doesn't necessarily mean that a person must sleep all that time, but time for relaxation as well as sleep should be planned.

A fourth principle that contributes to the quality of health is *Temperance*. What is temperance and how does it apply to health? Temperance is not overdoing any one thing—not overworking, overeating, doing anything that is not temperate. There are many instances in one's everyday experiences when intemperance may creep in; guarding against these is wise.

One of the strongest temptations that man has to encounter is appetite. Overeating is a common fault among the American people. Eating the wrong food is one of the causes of ill health. If the appetite is allowed to rule, the mind will not be in control. Hospitals are full of sick people, many of whom have not practiced the principle of healthful eating and have brought illnesses upon themselves. Because of lack of control of appetite, too many people torture the 30 feet of intestine with 3 inches of tongue.

A fifth great principle of health is *Abstinence*. Abstain from alcoholic beverages, coffee, tea, smoking, and drugs. They do harm to the body. Placing human beings under the control of alcohol results in the inability to think and eat intelligently. Alcohol, smoking, and drugs can cause great physical disabilities and ill health such as heart disease, cancer, and hepatitis. Abstinence also applies to overeating and a host of other activities when there is a tendency to excess. A worthwhile activity may be harmful when overindulged.

A further need is plenty of *Fresh Air* and *Sunlight* every day when possible. People are more dependent upon fresh air for the lungs than upon food for the stomach. Anyone who desires health and who would enjoy an active life should remember that he cannot have these without adequate circulation. Sunlight is an excellent source of vitamin D. While one should plan to enjoy fresh air and sunshine, one should be careful to avoid long periods of exposure to the sun to avoid burns and other possible complications.

All of these six principles should be incorporated in the daily health habits as a part of planning to be a healthy person.

A familiar saying is "one gets out of life what he puts into it." How much is the reader willing to put into his life right now? Enough to be in charge of "his body"? Enough to make wise decisions to eat each day those foods that will contribute to total well-being?

Even in trivialities, one has to make choices—a salad or a sandwich, an apple or a mango, a walk now or later. One's freedom is subject to the code which he has chosen to follow. Each one has the power to make choices, and each must live with the results of those choices.

The title of this chapter is, "You Are in Charge." Every person makes decisions, forms habits, establishes priorities that will affect the rest of his life. When success does not come his way, he has a tendency to blame circumstances, conditions, or even other people. But usually the responsibility is his own.

Values are seldom considered to be important. But values are vital to intelligent decision-making. Every person decides for himself where he wishes to go—sets standards and goals. He should not be satisfied until these standards and goals are met. He should eat to be a winner and stay well. Since the foods people eat have extreme effect upon the quality of daily life, one needs to remember that dieting is "mind over platter." Thinking positively about food and the worthwhile activities of the day is necessary.

To be in charge of one's self is being aware of possible problems to be solved. For example, some of the problems are:

1. Using food as a tranquilizer.
2. Nibbling whenever food is near.
3. Eating to be sociable.
4. Eating in response to the food's inviting aroma.
5. Using food to combat frustration, boredom, or loneliness.
6. Eating to keep awake.
7. Eating to resolve anger or hostility.
8. Using food as a reward.
9. Using food to counteract stress from overwork, illness, or serious loss.

Perhaps the reader may have one or more of these problems. If so, isolation of the problem, thinking of possible solutions, then choosing the most acceptable solution and following through will contribute to a sense of well-being.

What is the price tag to consider? The reader should think about his self-worth. The making of wise choices contributes to self-worth. When tempted to eat at the wrong time, or eat something he doesn't need, he should recall the title of this chapter, "You Are in Charge." A familiar saying is that one gets out of life what he puts into it. If the reader is willing to work out necessary changes in his life-style, then he is in charge. Wise choices require thinking, reasoning, common sense, and experience. Nothing is more self-rewarding than making choices that are worthwhile. The power to choose is what characterizes each individual. The choices made determine the results.

A person's success is subject to the code which he has chosen to follow. Everyone's privilege is to follow an intelligent mode of life and, by so doing, restore the principles of health to the body. Everyone needs to experience the rich reward that follows the making of wise choices. Man needs to learn the blessing of intelligent decisions in their fullness.

Chapter 9

The Advantages of Being a Vegetarian

Vegetarianism is a way of life. Eating what comes *naturally* is what vegetarianism is all about. Jean Mayer, M.D., a noted nutritionist at Harvard University, says, "Vegetarianism has three things going for it all at once. They are economics, health, and compassion."

Of these three ingredients, health is the main concern of the author; therefore, emphasis will be placed on health as related to vegetarianism.

Unfortunately, some confusion about nutrition exists in the minds of many people, especially among those who decide to adopt a vegetarian diet in a society of meat-eaters. An enormous amount of misinformation greatly compounds the problem. Protein is frequently the important issue with the quality and quantity of the protein questioned.

But, please accept these statements as demonstrated fact: the plant kingdom is a source of adequate nourishment. Every essential food substance for adequate nutrition is available from non-meat sources.

Dr. Mervyn G. Hardinge of the School of Public Health, Loma Linda University, in California writes: "From a nutritional point of view animal or vegetable proteins should not be differentiated. . . . The adequacy of protein intake depends not on the complexity of any single protein, but on the composition of the mixture of amino acids resulting from the breakdown of all the proteins in the meal."

The vegetarian who is a "pure" or total vegetarian excludes all animal products from the diet, i.e., meat, fish, poultry, milk, eggs, and cheese. A balanced diet for this individual needs careful attention to meet his nutritional needs. Plant foods do not contain a reliable amount of vitamin B_{12}. Milk and eggs are excellent sources, but the total vegetarian should consume fortified soybean milk, a vitamin B_{12} supplement, or nutritional yeast.

The vegetarian who is the lacto-ovo-vegetarian excludes all meat products including poultry, fish, and seafood. He eats dairy products such as milk, eggs, and cheese. For him the quality of protein is not a problem.

The "quality" of protein in plant foods is generally lower than that in animal protein. Protein *quality* is dependent upon the amounts and the availability of just eight of the twenty amino acids in protein. Animal protein contains these eight amino acids in the necessary amounts in the available forms, making a high-quality protein. On the other hand, plant proteins that are relatively low in some of the amino acids supplement one another when combined. Cereal grain proteins are relatively low in lysine, an essential amino acid; therefore, the addition of legumes will provide the needed lysine. Legumes, relatively low in methionine, an essential amino acid, may be combined with cereal grain to balance the amino acid supply. Thus, the combination results in high-quality protein.

While the meat-eater obtains his protein from meat, the vegetarian must obtain his protein from the vegetable kingdom. The secret for the vegetarian is simply choosing a wide variety of wholesome plant foods from the Basic Four Food Groups: whole grains, legumes (garbanzos, lentils, split peas, beans, and soybeans), nuts (cashews, walnuts, peanuts, Brazil nuts, almonds, pecans, and pine nuts), seeds (sunflower and sesame). These sources of protein combined with milk, eggs, cheese, vegetables, and fruits will provide a nourishing diet for the vegetarian. There is no single pattern in planning a vegetarian diet. One simply uses a wide variety of foods listed in the Basic Four Food Groups to provide the daily caloric requirements.

Soybeans are the source of many products that are manufactured and sold as substitutes for meats. Soybeans are processed by spinning and extrusion of the small, round bean, converting the product to soy protein, thread-like fibers, and forming realistic textures—known as synthetic products. Many meat-like products (meat analogues) are available in the health food store or market with beef-like, chicken-like, turkey-like, ham-like, bacon-like, bologna-like, salami-like, and cornbeef-like flavors and textures. These products are available as frozen or canned foods under various labels. A vegetarian "ground-beef-like" is also available—an excellent product from which the vegetarian can prepare "vegeburgers." "Vegeburger" should not be used directly from the can but should be combined with other ingredients to make a delicious vegetarian "burger." The recipe for making "vegeburgers" is in Section II of this volume.

Tofu, another soybean product, is a high-protein, cholesterol-free food made by solidifying soy milk. Tofu is relatively low in calories, a typical eight-ounce serving containing only 147 calories. Tofu is often used as a breakfast protein food to substitute for eggs. Combinations with such items as herbs, turmeric, parsley, onion, mushrooms, green pepper, tomatoes, and any other favorite vegetable make tofu a delight to eat.

All unrefined foods contain some protein: fruits, one to two grams per serving; vegetables, one to six grams per serving; bread, three and a half to four grams per serving; and eggs, seven grams per serving.

The following guidelines should be considered when changing to a vegetarian way of life:

1. Decrease the use of meat—increase the intake of legumes, whole grains, nuts, and meat substitutes.
2. Increase the intake of foods from the Basic Four Food Groups to supply adequate calories.
3. Increase the intake of breads and cereals to insure the B vitamins and iron.
4. Increase the intake of non-fat or low-fat milk products for protein and vitamin B_{12} when meat is deleted from the diet.

What are the advantages of the vegetarian diet over the typical American diet? A few worthwhile considerations include:

1. Lower blood cholesterol levels (fewer heart attacks).
2. Less possibility of contracting disease from animals (trichinosis, cancer, salmonellosis, and tuberculosis).
3. Increase in endurance (athletes).
4. Greater resistance to disease (cancer).
5. Less expensive.
6. Increase in fiber in the diet.
7. Longer shelf-life.
8. Less fat and less refined foods in the diet.
9. Less difficulty in controlling weight

Are vegetarians really healthier? Some of the recent studies of vegetarians versus meat-eaters have provided interesting results. An article in the *Journal of the American Medical Association*, July 2, 1982, states that "Eating meat raises systolic and diastolic blood pressure, and, conversely, a vegetarian diet lowers the pressure. And even though the meat-related pressure changes aren't gigantic or of an immediately life-threatening nature, one researcher believes they are important because differences in blood pressures between vegetarians and omnivores increase with advancing age. These blood-pressure differences may be caused by differences in the intake of fats and dietary fiber."

The *American Journal of Clinical Nutrition*, June, 1972, reports a study of the bone density of vegetarians versus meat-eaters in which vegetarians "were found to be less prone to osteoporosis (bone loss) than omnivores." Bone loss after age 40 is a major concern. It is estimated that 190,000 hip fractures occur yearly, at a cost of one billion dollars for acute care alone. Of these, two thirds are the result of osteoporosis.

A five-year study in 1965 on 5,700 Seventh-day Adventists in California was conducted by Loma Linda University. Examination of death certificates over a five-year period revealed that 98.8 percent showed the following results: Seventh-day Adventists lived 5–6 years longer in a given situation than non-Adventists in California, 85 percent had less heart disease, 70 percent less cancer, 68 percent less diseases of the respiratory system. A lower blood cholesterol level is achieved because of the practice of eating minimal animal fat. Much emphasis has been placed on decreasing the consumption of saturated fat. Here the vegetarian has an advantage over the meat-eater. With the abundant use of refined food, another problem has become evident, namely, the lack of fiber in the average American diet. Here again the vegetarian has the advantage by eating an abundance of fiber in fruits, grains, and vegetables.

From other studies and statistics, vegetarians have greater endurance against disease and a stronger endurance under physical stress. Athletes are able to endure much longer periods in a competition situation. A Swedish scientist gave nine athletes the same endurance test on a bicycle after the participants had been on a three-day (specific diet) program. Those on the high meat diet had an average endurance of 57 minutes. Those on a lower meat diet with some carbohydrates had an average endurance of 114 minutes. Those on the high carbohydrate diet had an average endurance of 167 minutes. Thus, the athletes on the lower meat diet with some carbohydrate had twice the endurance while those on the high carbohydrate diet had almost three times greater endurance than those on the high meat diet. The high carbohydrate diet was closely related to a vegetarian diet.

With the increase in population, animal food will be less available. Plants yield 800,000 calories per acre, but only 200,000 calories when the same plants are fed animals and man in turn eats the animal. To produce one pound of beef the animal must eat 7–8 pounds of grains.

Furthermore, the meat-eater is actually getting his food secondhand. In other words, animals eat the natural food, and humans eat the secondhand food.

Those who wish to cut back on meat consumption will want to choose carefully the kinds of cuts of meat to be eaten. There are restaurants that advertise gourmet meats without objectionable hormones and additives.

A few years ago vegetarians were viewed by many as "weirdos" or crusaders for carrot juice and peanut butter sandwiches. As a result, the vegetarian was embarrassed and kept the information about his eating practices "low key." Now, vegetarianism has become very popular and many meat-eaters are reducing or eliminating meat from their diets.

The author invites the reader to be adventurous and experiment with the recipes in Section II of this book. Many of the recipes are prepared from natural foods. Others use the meat analogues in one form or another. The recipes are simple to prepare and relatively low in cost.

The healthy vegetarian has a wholesome, varied, and interesting diet. He eats from the Basic Four Food Groups, using a wide variety of foods daily. He avoids refined foods, excess sugar, and excess fat. His diet is high in fiber since he eats fruits, vegetables, and unrefined foods. He eats whole grains in cereals and breads. These foods are delicious with natural flavors and contain large quantities of necessary nutrients for ultimate health.

To convert from a meat diet to a vegetarian diet is easier than most people think. One does not have to do all the changing at one time. By integrating vegetarian recipes with the daily meal plan, one can adapt one's eating habits without realizing much inconvenience.

A typical lacto-ovo-vegetarian menu:

Breakfast	Dinner	Supper
Orange Juice	Cottage Cheese Loaf	Vegeburger Sandwich
Brown Rice/Honey,	Baked Sweet Potato	with Tomato, Pickle,
Milk	Green Peas	Lettuce, Mayonnaise
Almonds	Cabbage Slaw/	Diced Figs
Canned or Fresh	Mayonnaise	Wheat Germ Cookies
Apricots	Rye bread/Margarine	Milk
Whole-Wheat Toast/	Milk	
Margarine		
Milk		

Legumes are easy to cook and are inexpensive. A "Crockpot" is a pot providing a simple method of preparation. These simple guidelines may be useful as the reader endeavors to make changes in eating habits.

Preparation of Dried Legumes

Dried legumes (beans, garbanzos, peas, and lentils) are an important, inexpensive source of protein in the diet. They are the same quality as cooked, canned legumes and can be prepared for a fraction of the cost of the canned product. There are several equally effective methods of cooking dried legumes, the only differences being the time and the facilities available.

Soaking and Cooking

1. In a strainer, rinse the measured amount of legumes to be cooked.

2. Place the legumes in a container and cover them with three to four times their volume of water.

3. Let stand (preferably in the refrigerator) overnight.

4. Transfer the legumes and the stock (the water used for soaking) to a saucepan. Bring the legumes and the stock to a boil. Lower heat and simmer until the legumes are the desired consistency, adding water as necessary.

Legumes	Dry Amount	Cooked Amount	Cooking Time (Soaked) (StoveTop)	Cooking Time (No Soaking) (Slow Cooker)	Cooking Time (No Soaking) (Pressure Cooker)
Garbanzo beans	1 cup	2¼ cups	4 hours	4–5 hrs 6–8 hrs	40–45 min
Great Northern beans	1 cup	2½ cups	2 hours	2–3 hrs 4–5 hrs	20–25 min
Lentils	1 cup	2⅔ cups	1 hour	1–2 hrs 2–3 hrs	10–15 min
Pinto beans	1 cup	2½ cups	2 hours	3–4 hrs 4–5 hrs	20–25 min
Red beans	1 cup	2½ cups	3 hours	3–5 hrs 5–7 hrs	30–35 min
White navy beans	1 cup	2½ cups	3 hours	3–4 hrs 5–7 hrs	30–35 min
Soybeans	1 cup	2½ cups	2 hours	2–3 hrs 4–5 hrs	20–25 min

Basic Roast

Choose 1 from *each* of the categories.

2 cups protein: kidney beans, lentils, garbanzos, meat analogues, tofu, cottage cheese, soy beans.

1 cup carbohydrate: dried whole-wheat bread crumbs, uncooked oatmeal, cooked brown rice, crushed cereal flakes, wheat germ.

Nuts, ½ cup, chopped or ground, raw: peanuts, cashews, almonds, walnuts.

Onion—1 chopped

Binding:
    4 tablespoons garbanzo flour
    6 tablespoons potato flour
    4 tablespoons soy flour
    ½ cup cooked oatmeal
    ½ cup cream of wheat
    4 egg whites

Liquid, 1½ cups as needed: tomato sauce or juice, broth from cooked or canned vegetables, or from canned meat analogues, milk, George Washington's Broth, McKay's Chicken-style broth.

Seasoning, ¼ teaspoon of one or more: sage, poultry seasoning, sweet basil, cumin, oregano, thyme, rosemary, Italian seasoning, bouquet garni, parsley (or 1 tablespoon chicken-like seasoning).

1 teaspoon salt or other seasoning salt (optional) or to taste

2 tablespoons oil or margarine

Sauté onion in oil. Add to other ingredients and press into lightly-oiled loaf pan, or shape into patties. Fry or bake and serve with a gravy.

Bake at 350° for 45 minutes (depending on thickness).
Serve with light gravy if desired.

Chapter 10
The Art of Vegetable Cookery

An old saying one often hears is that people "eat with their eyes," meaning that the food is so inviting they cannot resist eating. Color is important in making food attractive, and variety in color is easy to achieve with vegetables. Vegetables provide an array of colors to meet the needs of all occasions. For example, a menu consisting of an entrée with a baked potato is not strikingly beautiful, but the addition of colorful vegetables and garnishes will turn a drab plate into a piece of art. This goal is a challenge to any cook and should play an important part in menu planning. To accomplish this, there are helpful hints for purchasing, storing, preparing, cooking, combining, seasoning, and garnishing vegetables.

Purchasing top quality vegetables is very important. A knowledge of the grades and brands is needed to make wise choices among competing possibilities. Canned or frozen vegetables should be purchased by grades depending upon the uses to be made of them. High grades insure high quality. U. S. Grade A and Fancy Grade are the highest in quality—preferred in order to have the finished product colorful and tasty. The best grades insure the best flavor, uniformity of size, shape, color, tenderness, and represent the choice of the crop. Lower grades may be satisfactory for use in sauces, soups, or casseroles. Quantities and qualities that may be bought and used to the best advantage should be known in order to avoid long periods of storage.

Fresh vegetables reach a delicious high point at certain times of the year. Learning to take advantage of these in-season treats is wise. On the other hand, by using frozen or canned vegetables, variety at all times of the year may be achieved within the budget of the consumer. Harvesting vegetables for canning and freezing is a scientific project.

Color and nutrients are preserved carefully so there will not be any appreciable loss in food value and attractiveness.

When vegetables are purchased fresh, definite size, maturity, and color should be selected depending upon the use to be made of them. Immediately after taking purchases from the market to the home, proper cleaning and storage should be completed at once to conserve nutrients and freshness. Vegetables should be handled as little as possible and never soaked in the cleaning process. Vegetables should be peeled and cut as short a time before cooking as possible in order to keep the food values high. Trimming of vegetables may be necessary to remove damaged leaves or inedible material, but should be kept to a minimum. As a general rule, outer leaves, usually dark green, contain more nutrients than the inner leaves.

After the vegetables have been cleaned, they should be covered and stored at the appropriate temperature. Vegetables are very sensitive to handling. Preparing them is one of the greatest challenges of all cookery. However, if properly prepared, they will turn meals into something extra special. To achieve this goal, the chef or cook must be adventurous and dare to do something different.

Vegetables are very important in the diet because of the vitamins and minerals they provide. However, the nutrients the consumer actually receives depend on proper handling and preparation.

One of the greatest hazards in vegetable preparation is overcooking, which tends to ruin texture and color. Excess cooking makes vegetables turn dark in color, shrivel up in shape, and produce strong flavors that make them unappetizing. Vegetables should be cooked in as little water as possible in order to conserve the nutrients. The water should be saved for use in making soups or sauces. All vegetables should be covered (except cauliflower, broccoli, Brussels sprouts, and cabbage) to retain vitamins because oxidation destroys vitamins A and C. Cauliflower and potatoes are cooked to near-doneness before adding a minimum of salt to preserve the white color.

Vegetables vary in cooking time depending upon the specific vegetable, method of cookery, container used, and the maturity of the vegetable. The shorter the cooking period, the greater the vitamin retention. To shorten cooking time, vegetables may be cut, sliced, diced, or coarsely shredded. To insure the best flavor, texture, color, and food value, the vegetables should be cooked only until tender. Pressure cookers and microwave ovens contribute to shorter cooking periods and conservation of nutrients.

Cabbage, broccoli, and cauliflower should be cooked without a cover to preserve color and flavor. Overcooking should be avoided because it destroys vitamins and minerals and results in a strong flavor.

The use of bicarbonate of soda in vegetable cooking to retain color should be avoided because it tends to destroy vitamins and minerals. The best way to insure color and texture is to choose a top quality, fresh, frozen, or canned vegetable, use a small amount of water, cover the utensil during the cooking process, shorten the cooking time, and avoid rapid cooking at high temperatures.

Vegetable cookery is a challenging art in that there are many methods of preparation including steaming, frying, baking, braising, or even broiling. Variety in vegetable preparation may be obtained by combining one or more vegetables, using special seasonings, or adding sauces and dressings to enhance the flavor and the aroma for the enjoyment of the consumer.

One might vary sizes and shapes, such as cutting fresh vegetables in different ways, thereby adding a spark of delight to the plate. For example, celery or carrots may be sliced on the bias; potatoes, beets, carrots, cut waffle-style; carrots and beets, Julienne; carrots and parsnips, in circles; other vegetables may be cubed.

Vegetables are delicious on their own merits, but even irresistible when arranged in colorful combinations using special sauces or adding herbs. The finished flavor is important in the "selling" of the product. The use of vegetables upgrades menus for all occasions. In preparing menus, include vegetables of contrasting colors. The following suggestions give variety to menus:

1. Dark green *asparagus* may be arranged on a plate with pimento strips in the opposite directions, or served with an herb dressing of choice, or combined with whole kernel corn.

2. *Beets* cut Julienne may be flavored with orange juice for a delightful change.

3. *Broccoli* served with special sauces is most acceptable, such as baco-chips in a white sauce.

4. For added flavor, *Brussels sprouts* may be combined with celery, slivered almonds, grapes, green beans, or peas. Brussels sprouts may be served with special sauces, such as tomato sauce with grated American cheese, Hollandaise sauce, or sour cream.

5. To *cabbage* may be added celery seed, diced celery, or pearl onions.

6. *Carrots* combined with finely chopped parsley, celery crescents, or corn produce a delightful contrast. Pineapple or angel-flake coconut may be added for flavor.

7. *Celery* buttered with herbs added for flavor is a delightful change.

8. *Corn* may be combined with lima beans, kidney beans, zucchini, or peas.

9. *Green beans* may be enhanced by adding nuts, such as slivered almonds or filberts; or combined with pimento, mushrooms, onions, radishes, dill seed, or water chestnuts.

10. *Hominy* may be served with baco-chips or pearl onions.

11. *Onions* may be combined with peanuts.

12. *Parsnips* served with white sauce flavored with nutmeg are interesting.

13. *Peas* may be combined with cauliflower, new potatoes, mush-

rooms, celery crescents, pimento, chives, water chestnuts, or Julienne carrots.

14. *Spinach* may be spread with mayonnaise and shredded egg white and yolks in layers, cheese and eggs, Hollandaise sauce, or plain tartar sauce.

15. Cooked *sweet potatoes* may be served in orange cups, with apricots, marshmallows, or pecans added and baked slightly before serving.

16. *Tomatoes* may be combined with green pepper or stuffed with olives for added flavor.

17. *Turnips* may be combined with peas for contrast and flavor.

18. *Zucchini,* partly cooked and then stuffed with crumbs, cheese, parsley, and egg to hold ingredients together, sprinkled with cheese and browned before serving, is another suggestion.

All vegetables properly garnished add accent to the entire plate. In arranging foods on a plate or platter, sizes, shapes, and textures may be varied to produce line and form. Vegetables may be cut and arranged so that special decorating is unnecessary. Appeal to the appetite is keen, and the secret is simplicity in design, such as arranging spears of asparagus in various fashions on the bias, criss-cross, or like a fence. Such arrangements contribute to the overall psychological effects of balance, comfort, and mood. Each plate should be a beautiful, bright picture of the finest in color and combination. And the true artist knows when to stop, to avoid overdoing.

In summary, the art of vegetable cookery varies with the cook's pride in selecting, preparing, and serving tender, colorful, crisp, flavor-rich, and vitamin-laden vegetables. From asparagus to zucchini, nutrients rank high while the cost is low, and the calories are minimal.

Suggestions for Fresh Vegetable Preparation

Vegetable	Availability	Ways to Prepare	Suggested Seasonings and Accompaniments
Artichoke	January–June October–December	Simmered in water till tender	Lemon, dill, French dressing, mayonnaise, margarine
Asparagus	March–May	Boiled, baked, creamed	Lemon, butter, basil, thyme, mayonnaise, cheese sauce, margarine
Beets	All year	Boiled, baked, Harvard, raw, shredded	Lemon juice, clove, orange, caraway seed, green peppers, parsley, basil, thyme, mayonnaise
Broccoli	January–June	Boiled in water, raw flowerettes, oven baked, creamed	Flavored seeds, margarine, herbs, lemon, dill, cheese sauce, tartar sauce, mayonnaise
Brussels sprouts	October–April	Boiled whole or half, baked, stuffed, creamed	Caraway seed, basil, thyme, dill, lemon
Cabbage	All year	Baked, braised, cooked, creamed	Combine with other or raw vegetables, peppers, dill, lemon, pineapple, tomatoes, basil, sage, cheese sauce
Cauliflower	All year	Boiled, raw in salads, escalloped, creamed	Margarine flavored with dill, onion, sesame or poppy seed, lemon, cheese sauce, cheese, tomato, rosemary, egg and bread crumbs, curry, butter
Carrots	All year	Boiled, braised, shredded, raw or cooked, baked, creamed, vegetable stew	Orange, pineapple, sugar, clove, celery, minced onion, basil, egg sauce, marjoram, thyme

Vegetable	Availability	Ways to Prepare	Suggested Seasonings and Accompaniments
Celery	All year	Raw, sautéed, boiled, baked, stuffed, creamed	Basil, sage, margarine, mushrooms
Corn on cob	May–November	Boiled, roasted, baked	Green pepper, margarine, cream, escalloped, tomato, pimento
Corn, cut	May–November	Boiled, baked	Escalloped, tomato, cream, margarine, pimento
Eggplant	All year	Baked, boiled, fried, mashed, escalloped, breaded, stuffed	Cheese, oregano, dill, marjoram, thyme, tomato, onion
Green beans	All year	Boiled, creamed	Marjoram, rosemary, mushrooms, onion, nutmeg, thyme, parsley, dill seed, tarragon, lemon juice, slivered almonds, tomatoes, cheese sauce, basil, sage
Greens	Some variety all year	Boiled	Marjoram, mayonnaise, lemon
Kohlrabi	May–November	Boiled, baked, creamed	Margarine, lemon, tomato sauce, cheese
Lima beans	All year	Boiled, creamed	Pimento, mushrooms, onions, nutmeg, thyme, sage, tarragon, lemon juice, tomatoes, parsley, green peppers, cheese, basil
Mushrooms	All year	Simmered, creamed, stuffed, sautéed	Oregano, thyme, margarine, rosemary
Okra	All year	Baked, boiled, breaded	Tomatoes, mayonnaise, creamed
Onions, dry	All year, peak May–Nov.	Sautéed, boiled, baked, creamed, buttered	Margarine, cheese, thyme, marjoram, oregano

Vegetable	Availability	Ways to Prepare	Suggested Seasonings and Accompaniments
Parsnips	All year	Baked, glazed, vegetable stew, sautéed, mashed	Margarine, parsley, dill, onion, lemon
Peas	All year, peak April–May	Boiled, creamed	Dill, mint, mushrooms, celery, cheese sauce, basil, marjoram, thyme, sage, margarine, cream, carrots
Peppers	All year	Stuffed, diced, chopped, boiled, baked	Rice, corn, fillings, margarine, tomatoes
Potatoes, white	All year	Baked, boiled, stuffed, vegetable stew, escalloped, creamed, mashed	Cheese, onion, tomato, parsley, sage, margarine, rosemary
Spinach	All year, peak spring & fall months	Creamed, boiled	Cheese sauce, lemon, onion, basil, celery, marjoram, thyme, rosemary, mayonnaise
Squash, summer, includes Italian crookneck, etc.	Some varieties all year	Baked, sautéed, boiled	Margarine, onion, garlic, peppers, tomato, marjoram, thyme, sage
Squash, winter	Some varieties all winter	Baked, mashed	Glaze of orange, lemon, pineapple, sugar, cloves, nutmeg, sage, margarine
Sweet potato	All year	Baked, boiled, glazed, mashed	Clove, pineapple, sugar, honey, orange, lemon, caramel, margarine
Tomatoes	All Year	Stewed, baked, boiled, escalloped, creamed, breaded, stuffed	Basil, oregano, sage, margarine
Turnips and Rutabaga	All year	Boiled, baked, creamed	Clove, ginger, onion, caraway, margarine, sage, rosemary

Chapter 11

Beverages—What Are You Drinking?

Beverages present an effective way of introducing fluid into the body. They may be drinks of different kinds and flavored with various substances—some of which may be harmful. Tea, coffee, and chocolate contain a stimulant which affects the nervous system and the heart. In addition, they contain tannin, an astringent which retards the process of digestion.

The most popular beverage in this country is coffee. Even some young children drink coffee regularly. Statistics show that the average user drinks from three to four cups of coffee each day. Many, of course, drink much more. Why is coffee such a popular beverage? A few replies from coffee drinkers include: "It gives me a pick-up," "It makes me feel more alert," "I can think better," or "I just feel better."

Over half of the world's coffee is used in the United States, and caffeine consumption is not limited to coffee, tea, and chocolate. Actually, caffeine is found in most all cola beverages, and these are consumed in large quantities. In fact, the consumption of cola beverages is now greater than 30 gallons per capita per year.

Why the concern regarding coffee consumption? Caffeine beverages are stimulants that have exhilarating effects upon the body. They excite nerves around the heart to increased action, and produce short-lived energy to the entire system. Since the results are so stimulating, many people believe that drinking beverages that contain caffeine is beneficial. However, these beverages provide negligible nutrients. The effect of caffeine on the body is mainly to trigger the release of sugar into the blood, providing fuel for immediate use, thereby giving a sense of renewed energy. However, this energy may be considered to be "borrowed" energy.

Caffeine stimulates the nervous system, and, although it may remove a sense of fatigue, it cheats the body by producing sleep-lessness. The principles governing energy would suggest that one cannot get something for nothing. How can stimulation produced by a drug like caffeine, secure any energy except at a corresponding expense?

Information from an article in the *Journal of the American Medical Association*, "The Role of Drugs in Production of Gastroduodenal Ulcer," 187:418, 1964, indicates this "new" energy or stimulation is followed by a "let-down" and a period of fatigue characterized by decreased efficiency and alertness while the body attempts to recuperate from loss of the "used-up" energy. The continued and generous use of caffeine beverages may result in headache, wakefulness, palpitation of the heart, indigestion, trembling, and other effects such as two distinct actions on gastric secretion: direct stimulation of the secreting cells, and increased activity of other stimulating substances that may be present, such as alcohol and meat extracts.

Studies have shown a correlation between excessive coffee drinking and coronary heart disease. Most cardiologists have found coffee to be a stressful substance, and have observed that the continual use of a drug which is prone to be habit-forming causes the body to become so accustomed to its presence that when the drug is discontinued certain undesirable effects result. Caffeine is just such a drug, and anyone attempting to stop after a long period of intake may suffer withdrawal symptoms. Caffeine also stimulates the production of stomach acids, which may produce heartburn.

In 1972 at Loma Linda University, in California, a study was done to determine the reaction of spiders to caffeine. Spiders are well-known for their production of beautiful, perfectly symmetrical webs. When they are given caffeine, the webs are grossly distorted. Only after many hours have passed can the spiders again produce a perfect web.

Decaffeinated coffees are very popular and highly advertised. But they contain substances other than caffeine that may be harmful. Most decaffeinated coffees have 90–96 percent of the caffeine removed, but some of the other ingredients are:

1.25% Cafferal
12% Fat
12% Tannic acid

While cafferal is a volatile acid that contributes flavor and aroma, tannic acid, also present, tends to check digestion and to retard absorption of nutrients.

Of the three popular caffeine beverages, tea, coffee, and "coke," tea is considered the least harmful. The caffeine-tannin in tea is in ratio of one to three. Tea is a stimulant, and contains two grams of tannin in the average cup. Coffee and tea are not healthful beverages, and the author urges the reader to discontinue their use.

Chocolate and cocoa contain less of the objectionable qualities than tea and coffee. However, if a person is a "chocoholic," he could be getting a significant amount of various chemicals. Martin Rehfuss in his book, *Indigestion,* p. 492, reports that cocoa and chocolate contain theobromine, a small amount of caffeine, a small amount of tannin, and a small amount of fat.

All brands of cocoa made according to the instructions on the box contain more tannin per cup than is usually found in a cup of tea, according to *Consumer's Research Bulletin,* February, 1946. Chocolate and cocoa delay digestion and require a relatively long period in the stomach. Another concern when using chocolate and cocoa is the amount of sugar needed to make them palatable. The use of sugar is greatly increased in this manner.

According to *Larousse Gastronomique, an Encyclopedia of Food, Wine, and Cookery,* 1961, the following statement is made concerning cocoa: "Cocoa, among its principal aromatics, contains various alkaloids, the most important of which are theobromine and caffeine. Cocoa, which contains about 17 percent of nitrogenous matter, 25 percent fats, and 38 percent carbohydrates, has an important food value and, above all, a stimulating action which produces an immediate result, even before it has time to be assimilated."

Here are some interesting findings relative to cocoa and chocolate:

	Theobromine Content	Caffeine
Cocoa: 1 cup (5 oz) beverage	70 mg.	7 mg.
Baking chocolate: 5 oz.	125–550 mg.	13 mg.
Chocolate bars: 3½ oz.	180–550 mg.	18 mg.

The use of cola drinks and other carbonated beverages has greatly increased in recent years, and the consumption of such soft drinks has become firmly entrenched in the American style of living. Today over five billion dollars are spent annually on soft drinks. The average American is drinking about 400 (8-ounce) bottles a year, including cola beverages. Soft drinks contain about ten to fifteen percent sugar. An eight-ounce bottle of an average carbonated beverage, or cola drink, contains about 100 calories and few, if any, nutrients.

The caffeine content of selected beverages, according to *Consumer Reports,* October, 1981, is:

		Caffeine
1 cup drip coffee, 5 oz.	146 mg.	"
1 cup percolated coffee	110 mg.	"
1 cup instant coffee (regular)	53 mg.	"
1 cup decaffeinated coffee	2 mg.	"
1 cup tea (5-min. brew)	20–50 mg.	"
12 oz. canned ice tea	22–36 mg.	"
12 oz. can Coca-Cola	34 mg.	"
12 oz. can Dr. Pepper	38 mg.	"
12 oz. can diet Dr. Pepper	37. mg.	"
12 oz. can Mr. Pibb	52 mg.	"
12 oz. can Mountain Dew	52 mg.	"
12 oz. can Tab	44 mg.	"

12 oz. can Pepsi-Cola	37 mg.	"
12 oz. can R.C. Cola	36 mg.	"
12 oz. can Diet Rite Cola	34 mg.	"
1 oz. milk chocolate	6 mg.	"
6 oz. cocoa beverage (water mix)	10 mg.	"

Many people have difficulty in believing the amount of caffeine contained in many common beverages. One must read the labels. However, if the word "cola" is a part of the trade name, the caffeine content need not be shown on the label. The FDA allows manufacturers to add caffeine to soft drinks, up to 0.02 percent by weight. This is about half the amount of caffeine in a cup of coffee. *Added caffeine is listed on the ingredients label.**

As an alternative to caffeine-containing beverages, there are cereal beverages, some with delicious flavor, especially some that are prepared in Europe. Some herb teas, such as peppermint and orange, are also delicious and popular.

Fruit juices are rich in nutrients because they furnish minerals and vitamins. These juices are available in various combinations inviting to the eye and appealing to the palate. Surprisingly, pineapple juice combined with tomato juice in equal proportions makes a delicious and refreshing drink. Many fruit juice combinations are available. Pure juices are recommended in the place of juice beverages. Most juice beverages contain little juice and usually a substantial amount of sugar.

Chapter 12
Eat for a Happy Heart

Heart disease is the number one killer in America today. Doctors are urging people to change their diets to avoid clogging blood vessels with fatty substances.

There is perhaps no part of the human anatomy that is more vital to well-being than the organs of circulation, which include the heart, arteries, veins, and capillaries. Health is the free and unhampered circulation of pure blood through a sound organism. As long as this stream of blood can reach every cell and tissue of the body, the individual is more likely to continue life for a longer time, for each cell and organ depends for its life on the blood stream. There are some 6,000 miles of blood vessels in the body, yet the exchange of blood in the most distant parts requires but a few seconds.

Since heart diseases claim thousands of deaths each year, a great public interest has been awakened in causes and prevention.

Fatty items in the diet are largely responsible for heart disease. However, fat alone is not the whole problem. Other faulty habits— overeating, irregular or late meals, inadequate diets—all have a definite bearing upon disturbances of the circulatory system. Certain types of fat in the diet cause a condition known as atherosclerosis, which is a narrowing of the blood vessels caused by thickening of the arterial walls. A definite relationship exists between certain types of fat in the diet and blood cholesterol.

Fats and Cholesterol

Fats and cholesterol are so closely associated that they will be discussed together in this chapter. They are both major factors in coronary heart disease. Cholesterol is a fatty substance found in foods. Many studies show that cholesterol levels can be reduced nearly to normal with diet and drugs. Some families are prone to high cholesterol levels; if so, they should give special attention to the information in this chapter. An important goal is to reduce cholesterol in the diet and prevent its collection in the arteries.

The amount and kind of fat found in animals and animal products should be considered. The use of animal fat increases the risk of hardening of the arteries, and it has been said that one is as old as his arteries!

Foods that are high in cholesterol or saturated fat should be avoided. These foods include egg yolks, organ meats, sweet breads, regular ground beef, spare ribs, bacon, sausage, cold cuts, heavily marbled and fatty meats, whole milk (3.5–4 percent fat), cheese, butter, cream, regular and non-dairy ice cream, ice milk, lard, shortening, meat drippings, gravies, egg noddles, most canned soups, chocolate, and coconut.

Since these foods are high in cholesterol, one should substitute foods of moderate or low cholesterol or low saturated fat wherever possible. Such foods include lean meats, skim milk (less than 1 percent fat), low-fat cottage cheese, yogurt, nuts (except cashews and macadamia), breads (except egg or cheese breads), crackers (except cheese crackers), packaged dehydrated soups, bouillon, sherbet, and cocoa.

Foods with little or no cholesterol or saturated fat may be used generously. These include: vegetables (fresh, frozen, or canned), fruits (fresh, frozen, or canned), egg whites, gelatin, all cereals, legumes (beans), rice, macaroni, spaghetti, flour, and fruit ice.

Where the use of meat is regarded as essential, the following changes should be considered:

1. Serve less meat.
2. Reduce size of meat portions.
3. Avoid processed meats high in saturated fat: hot dogs, luncheon meats, salami, sausage, bologna, hamburger.
4. Avoid organ meats and shellfish.
5. Choose lower-fat cuts and cuts low in marbling. Trim well!
6. Remove skin on poultry.
7. Avoid duck and goose.

Low cholesterol cooking is largely a matter of approach. Foods may be seasoned with herbs that help to bring out the best in flavors. Cooking with a bit of flair, doing something special, planning in advance will contribute to eating "for your heart's delight." When the essential fatty acid intake is low or lacking, the transport of cholesterol is retarded and cholesterol accumulates in the blood serum and walls of blood vessels. The same reaction occurs when the cholesterol intake is high.

Dr. Castelli emphasized in an article published in the *Medical Tribune Report,* April 8, 1981, that in the treatment of heart disease, "The key factor is total intake of dietary fat, which poses both a carcinogenic and cardiological risk." He said in an interview, "Cardiologists have moved away from an early emphasis on low dietary polyunsaturated to total reduction of fat intake." The literature on the animal studies indicates that there may be little choice between polyunsaturated and saturated fat, but there are major choices if one considers high- and low-fat diets. Dr. Castelli continued by saying, "Epidemiologically, countries with the highest incidence of breast cancers tend to have high fat diets."

"Jack Sprat could eat no fat," is one way of ensuring a low cholesterol intake. The diet does not need to be boring even though some might think so. It is time to put that myth to rest. Omitting butter, egg yolks, cream, and animal fats from cooking does not automatically result in the kitchen's symphony being off-key or full of flat notes. The ever-increasing list of low-fat products on the market comes to the aid of the cook who is determined that family and friends eat well while making wise choices.

Markets and Labels

Labeling is the method used by the food industry to acquaint consumers regarding the contents of the product. The consumer will soon realize the importance of understanding the label. For example, on the label for margarine, triglycerides and monoglycerides are listed in the ingredients. These could be from either an animal or a vegetable source. To insure unsaturated fat, the label should read *vegetable* triglycerides and monoglycerides. Most cheeses are high in butter fat. Skim milk or partially skim cheeses are an acceptable substitute. Mozzarella, hoop, ricotta, uncreamed cottage cheese, and low-fat cheeses may be used because of the reduced fat content. Yellow cheeses, cream cheeses, and creamed cottage cheese should be used sparingly because of the high fat content.

Plain yogurt may replace sour cream. Imitation creamers are available; for example, Mocha Mix, which contains no cholesterol. Most imitation milks, creamers, and whips replace butter fat with a vegetable fat, usually a coconut oil. However, studies indicate that coconut oil raises serum cholesterol in humans. Since coconut oil is one of the very few vegetable oils that is highly saturated, products containing coconut oil should be avoided. Lard and solid shortenings should be replaced by liquid vegetable oils, such as corn oil or soybean oil. Eggs are high in cholesterol and should be used sparingly. Egg whites may be used as a substitute for whole eggs.

The total caloric intake should be distributed as follows: 12 percent from protein, 30 percent from fat, and 58 percent from carbohydrates, as recommended by the 1977 Senate Select Committee on Nutrition and Human Needs.

The previous considerations in this chapter have been concerned with a decrease in fat and cholesterol. The next item to be discussed is the Committee's recommendation to increase fiber in the diet.

Fiber

Fiber is another important factor in coronary heart disease, but a factor that should be *increased,* not *decreased.* What is fiber and why is it important in the diet? People may recognize fiber by its old name, roughage or bulk. What are the advantages of fiber in the diet? Fiber . . .

1. decreases food intestinal transit time,
2. increases excretion of fatty acids,
3. lowers serum cholesterol.

Fiber is plant residue and makes up the cell walls in plants, forms part of the roots, stem, leaves, and fruit. Humans do not digest fiber, but its presence in the diet is thought to make a major contribution to total health. Added vegetable fiber absorbs and holds water, increases stool mass, and decreases transit time of intestinal content. Researchers are investigating the possible effects of fiber on the serum cholesterol. A high fiber diet may help to lower the serum cholesterol level.

Dietary fiber refers to all foods that reach the large intestine essentially unchanged. In the *British Journal of Nutrition* 7:98, 1953, the following was noted regarding fiber and food intestinal transit time: "Brown bread mixed with barium left the stomach and passed through the small intestine more rapidly, and left the colon 24 hours sooner than a similar amount of white bread."

Of the foods consumed in the U.S., unfortunately, 86 percent are nonfiber foods: 23 percent meat and eggs, 18 percent fats and oils, 17 percent refined cereals, 17 percent sugar, and 11 percent milk. The fiber foods usually amount to only 14 percent, consisting of 8 percent fruits and vegetables, 3 percent whole grain, and 3 percent legumes.

The second advantage of dietary fiber is the increased excretion of fatty acids. Fiber increases the excretion of fatty acids, bile acids, and sterols as noted in the *American Journal of Clinical Nutrition* 11:42, 1962. A study in rats showed that excretion was increased when cellulose was added to the diet (*Arch Biochemistry Biophysics,* 76:367, 1958). Another observation showed that bile salts and acids are more readily absorbed in vegetable fibrous tissue, (*Biochimica Biophysia Acta* 152:165, 1968).

The third advantage of dietary fiber is the lowering of serum cholesterol. *Lancet* 2:303, 1963, noted a study done on 26 male volunteers. When the subjects were fed rolled oats, the serum cholesterol levels were reduced from 251 mg percent to 223 mg percent, on the average, in three weeks. Another study showed that in ten girls, ages 10–12, 100g of cellulose per day reduced the serum cholesterol levels from 226mg to 170mg (*Nature* 232:554, 1971).

An interesting fact is that food preparation affects fiber content. Toasting, browning, or baking tend to increase fiber content. Sautéed vegetables have more fiber than boiled. Steaming tends to spare pectins and gum, both of which are water-soluble fibers.

Dr. Hugh Trowell, *Life and Health,* October, 1972, "Coronary Heart Disease and Fiber in Food," p. 22–23, classified certain foods in relation to fiber content by caloric intake, as follows:

Foods rich in fiber (8–15 gm. per 1000 calories): leguminous seeds, fully mature; beans, peas, lentils, some nuts. Young seeds have considerably less fiber content.

Foods with moderate amount of fiber (5–8 gm. per 1000 calories): all cereals and flours, whole grains. Examples: rice, corn, rye, barley, wheat, millet. Starchy roots and tubers, such as potatoes or yams, contain as much fiber as wheat in proportion to their caloric content.

Fruits and vegetables have 0.5–2 gm. per 100 gm. weight.

Foods depleted of fiber: corn meal (60% extraction) = 2 gm per 1000 calories; polished rice = 0.6 gm. per 1000 calories; other refined or highly processed food products.

Fiber-free foods: fats and oils, spreads, eggs, milk, sugar, meat, fish, and all beverages.

If one eats a sweet, starchy diet, one tends to put on weight and have poor elimination. When adequate fiber is ingested, the problem of constipation is largely solved.

Whole-grain cereals have fiber. Vegetables and fruits have fiber. Apple peel and celery are excellent sources of fiber. Bran is sometimes added to bread and cereals, thereby increasing the fiber content. Rice bran is high in fiber; lentils also are an excellent source of fiber. A wide variety of fruits and vegetables should be chosen and refined foods avoided. Natural sources are selected for best results.

Many people do not understand the function of fiber in the digestive system. They tend to think of fiber merely as a "laxative" to use when symptoms of constipation occur. Fiber also has the ability to clean all the convolutions in the intestines. Fiber removes toxins and wastes deposited in the intestines from all the systems of the complex organisms. By adding fiber to the daily eating pattern, one will be amazed at the results.

To assist in choosing fiber foods, the table on the following pages is provided.

Fiber Content of Some Common Foods on an Average Serving Basis

The following table shows the content of fiber in various foods.

Beans, cooked, ½ C:	grams	Cereals, ¾ C dry:	grams
Cowpeas	1.4	Bran-All	3.5
Garbanzos	2.5	Bran flakes, 40%	1.0
Lentils	1.0	Bran and raisin	1.05
Lima, baby	1.6	Cheerios	0.23
Lima, green	1.8	Corn flakes	0.10
Red kidney	1.5	Oatmeal	0.30
Snap, green	0.6	Post Toasties	0.10
Soybeans	1.1	Rice Krispies	—
Wax, yellow	0.5	Rice, puffed	0.10
White	1.5	Wheaties	0.38
		Wheat, puffed	0.15
Breads 1 slice:	grams	Wheat, shredded	0.50
		Wheat, Chex	0.90
Boston, brown	0.2		
Bran, raisin	0.5		
Corn	0.2	Cereals ½ C cooked:	grams
Cracked wheat	0.1	Corn grits	.15
Pumpernickel	0.4	Cream of Wheat, quick	.05
Raisin, plain	0.2	Farina	.10
Roman meal	0.3	Malt-o-Meal	.07
Rye, American	0.1	Oats, rolled	.25
White	tr.	Ralston	.45
Whole-wheat	0.4	Rice, brown	.13
		Rice, white	.07
Other Breads and Rolls:	grams		
		Others, ½ C cooked:	grams
Danish pastry	0.1		
Muffin	0.1	Macaroni	.05
Pancake	0.1	Noodles, egg	.10
Roll, white	0.1	Spaghetti	.05
Roll, whole-wheat	0.6	Millet	1.60
Tortilla, corn	0.3	Whole-wheat	1.40
Waffle	0.1	Wheat, cracked	.50

Nuts, ½ oz:	grams
Almonds, 5 nuts	0.4
Brazil, 4 med. nuts	0.3
Cashew, 6–8 nuts	0.2
Filberts, 10–12 nuts	2.3
Peanuts, no skin, 1T	0.2
Pecans, 12 halves	0.3
Pistachios, 30 nuts	0.3
Walnuts, English 1T.	0.3

C-cup   lg-large   sm-small
T-tablespoon   m-medium

Vegetables, ½ C cooked:	grams	Fruits, raw or fresh:	grams
Asparagus	0.5	Apple, 1 med.	1.5
Bean sprouts	0.4	Apricots, 2–3 med.	0.6
Beets	0.7	Bananas, 1 sm. (6″)	0.5
Beet greens	1.3	Blueberries, ⅝ C	1.5
Broccoli	1.5	Boysenberries, ⅘ C	2.7
Brussels sprouts	1.6	Cantaloupe, ¼ melon	0.3
Cabbage	0.7	Cherries, ½ C	0.2
Cabbage, raw, ½ C	0.4	Dates, 5	1.1
Carrots	0.8	Figs, 2 lg	1.2
Carrots, raw 1 lg.	1.0	Fruit cocktail, ½ C	0.4
Cauliflower	0.5	Grapefruit, ½ med.	0.2
Cauliflower, raw ½ C	0.5	Grapes, 22 med. (⅔ C)	0.6
Celery	0.3	Honeydew, 2″ wide slice	0.9
Celery, raw, 1 outer stalk	0.3	Nectarine, 2 med.	0.4
Chard, Swiss	0.6	Orange, 1 med.	0.8
Collards	0.8	Peach, 1 med.	0.6
Corn	0.7	Pear, ½ med.	1.4
Cucumber, with skin, ½ m	0.3	Persimmon, 1 med.	1.6
Eggplant	0.9	Pineapple, ¾ C.	0.4
Lettuce, butterhead, 1 C	0.5	Plums, 2 med.	0.4
Lettuce, Romaine, 1 C	0.7	Prunes, 2 lg.	0.4
Lettuce, iceberg, 1 C	0.5	Raspberries, ½ C	2.0
Lettuce, leaf, 1 C	0.7	Strawberries, 10 lg. (¾ C)	1.3
Mustard greens	0.9	Tangerine, 1 lg., 2 sm.	0.5
Okra	1.0	Watermelon, ½ circle	
Onions	0.5	slice, 1″ thick	1.8
Onions, raw, 1 T	0.1		
Parsnips	2.0		
Peas	1.5		
Peppers, green	0.7		
Peppers, green, raw, 1 lg.	1.4		
Potatoes	0.6		
Pumpkin	1.5		
Radish, raw, 10 sm.	0.7		
Rutabaga	1.1		
Spinach	0.5		
Squash, summer	0.6		
Squash, winter	1.8		
Sweet potatoes	0.9		
Tomatoes	0.6		
Tomatoes, raw, 1 med.	0.8		
Yams	0.9		

Bowes and Church. *Food Values of Portions Commonly Used*, J. B. Lippincott Co., PA and Toronto. 11th edition, 1970.

Other Factors

Salt is another important factor in heart disease. The general recommendation is that salt consumption should be lowered by 50 to 85 percent. To achieve this goal one should cook sparingly with salt, and not add salt at the table. Given an excess of salt in the diet, the "taste" for this seasoning increases. Many people never bother to taste the food until the salt shaker has been shaken vigorously over the plate.

Salt is a chemical compound made up of 40 percent sodium and 60 percent chlorine. Although the body must have sodium, most people eat much more than is needed. Sodium in salt tends to contribute to high blood pressures in some people. Reducing the use of salt and other products that contain sodium can help reduce the amount of medication needed. By limiting sodium intake, some people can lower blood pressure without taking medication.

Sodium occurs naturally in food, about one third again as much is often added either in the processing of foods or in the kitchen as the food is prepared. The average person consumes about two teaspoons of table salt each day. This amount, approximately 4,000 mg., greatly exceeds the needs of the body. Only 200 mgs are necessary for the body to function properly.

Caffeine is still another factor in coronary heart disease. Two separate studies reported in the *New England Journal of Medicine* (April 17 and June 16, 1983), suggest that caffeine may not only present a problem for some individuals who may already have heart disease, but also may be involved in the development of the disease. Caffeine has been found to contribute to the irregular heart beats of those who had pre-existing heart disease.

Nicotine. Cigarette smokers have 2–3 times the incidence of heart disease as do non-smokers.

Obesity is another factor to be considered in coronary heart disease. Obesity increases the chances for a heart attack by 10 to 13 percent for those 20 percent overweight; and at 30–40 percent overweight the chance of a fatal heart attack increases from 30 to over 40 percent. A possible cause of being overweight is excessive calories ingested, with little or no exercise. If exercise is a key to improving cardiovascular health, what type of exercise is most likely to be effective? Many kinds of exercise are available; however, just walking briskly for 30 minutes is very helpful.

Stress and Tension may be important factors affecting coronary heart disease. Stress, overwork, and many other facets of today's fast-moving world are of major concern. Stress and tension are discussed in Chapters 16 and 17. Everyone should take time to relax. The heart is a muscle and rebels against overwork.

Sugar is a dietary element that should be reduced. Excessive refined carbohydrates are a major contribution to obesity. One should achieve and maintain normal weight—a little on the lean side is recommended. Fruits are recommended for desserts in place of pie, cake, or ice cream.

Alcohol is a contributing factor to coronary heart disease. In addition to its devastating effects, it contributes calories with minimal nutrition.

Fats in Cream and Cream Substitutes

The following list shows the percent of fat in cream and cream substitutes:

	Percent		Percent
Cream		*Sweetened*	
Whole Milk	3.0– 3.8	Dry Powders	
Half-and-Half	10.0–12.0	Dream Whip	37.8
Cream		Lucky Whip	40.4
Light Cream	16.0–22.0	Semi-Solid	
Whipping Cream	30.0–38.0	Cool Whip	24.5
Cultured Sour	12.0–20.0		
Cream		Whipped: aerosol can	
Unsweetened		Ditto	19.0
Dry Powders		Reddi Whip	26.1
Coffee-Mate	1.9	Rich's Whip	18.5
Cremora	1.8	Topping	
N-Rich	1.2	*Artificially sweetened (dry powder)*	
Pream	3.4	D'Zerta Low	55.0
Liquid		Calorie Whipped	
Coffee-Rich	10.3	Topping	
Soured, Semi-solid			
Imo	19.8		
Zevo, imitation	19.4		
sour cream			

References from "Fatty Acid Composition and Total Lipid of Cream and Cream Substitutes," *The American Journal of Clinical Nutrition*, 22:4, April, 1969, pp 458–463.

Cholesterol Listings

The following list shows comparative levels of cholesterol or saturated fat in various foods:

Foods High in Cholesterol or Saturated Fat

Egg yolks
Organ meats
Sweet breads
Regular ground beef
Spare ribs, bacon, sausages
Cold cuts of all kinds
Heavily marbled and fatty meats

Whole milk, cheese, and butter
Creams, regular and non-dairy
Ice cream and ice milks
Lard and shortening
Meat drippings and gravies
Egg noodles
Most canned soups
Chocolate and coconut

Foods Moderate in Cholesterol or Saturated Fat

Lean meats
Regular cottage cheese

Foods Low in Cholesterol or Saturated Fat

Skim milk
Low-fat cottage cheese and yogurt
Peanut butter, margarine
Nuts (except cashews and
  macadamia)
Breads (except egg or cheese
  breads)

Crackers (except cheese crackers)
Packaged dehydrated soups
Bouillon
Sherbet
Cocoa

Foods with NO Cholesterol or Saturated Fat

Vegetables—fresh, frozen, or
  canned
Fruits—fresh, frozen, or canned
Egg whites, gelatin
All cereals and legumes (beans)
Rice, macaroni, and spaghetti
Flour, fruit ice

Corn oil, safflower oil
Corn oil, safflower tub-type
  margarines
Soft drinks
Pure sugar, honey
Olives, pickles, salt, herbs

In summary, to reduce risk of heart disease, the following dietary changes are suggested:

1. Skim off fats from soups and stews.
2. Braise in small amounts of water instead of oil.
3. Use newer types of cooking ware; example, Teflon.
4. Experiment with recipes to reduce total fat.
5. Limit use of nuts, olives, foods already salted.
6. Avoid baked goods and candies high in saturated fat and/or cholesterol.
7. Bake, broil, and simmer instead of frying foods.
8. Substitute natural foods for prepared and packaged foods.
9. Reduce amount of salt used on the table and in cooking.
10. Increase consumption of whole grains, fruits, vegetables, and legumes.
11. Substitute fruits for pastries.
12. Substitute cornstarch in the place of a mixture of butter and flour in preparing sauces and gravies.

In addition, the following suggestions may help in making necessary changes so that one may live with a "happy heart":

1. Keep the weight down to ideal level.
2. Keep cholesterol intake under 300 mg. per day.
3. Keep total fat down to 30 percent of the calories.
4. Keep saturated fat down to under 10 percent of the calories.
5. Keep sugar intake down to 5 percent of the calories or about 6–7 teaspoons per day.
6. Keep the salt intake down to 1 teaspoon per day.
7. Keep the use of fruit, vegetables, and whole grains to the suggested meal plan for each day.
8. Keep exercising, every day.
9. Keep a high-fiber food usage.
10. Keep caffeine out of the diet.

Chapter 13

Dietary Factors in Cancer Prevention

Cancer is the second greatest killer in the United States. The very word, "Cancer," is frightening. Most of us know someone who has had cancer and fear that some day we, too, may have the dreaded disease. To be knowledgeable about the causes of cancer is one of the best defenses against it. Studies indicate that 80 percent of cancer can be prevented and that diet is a contributing factor that definitely makes a tremendous difference. Other studies show that 40 percent of cancer in men and 60 percent in women are connected to poor choices in nutrition. The most desirable approach to disease control is prevention. This is especially true for neoplasia, which is the development of new, abnormal tissue, such as a tumor or growth.

Since cancer is an international problem, many cooperative studies done in various countries have revealed pertinent information on key etiologic factors. In comparative studies on the incidence of cancer in the United States and in other parts of the world, certain cultural practices have been considered to be advantageous in preventing cancer. For example, studies indicate that Japan is a low-risk country, and many other parts of Asia fall into this category. Africa also has a low-risk record. The United States, however, is a high-risk country. The interesting and appalling fact to note is that when an immigrant from a low-risk country migrates to the United States and adapts to Western eating habits, he may individually change from a low-risk to a high-risk category.

When the eating habits of various cultures are compared, some interesting observations may be made. The United States, with a high-risk factor for cancer, is known for the consumption of rich, refined foods, and animal fats. The fat intake apparently is of concern since a high-animal-fat intake produces an increase in bile acids.

Studies indicate that when bile acids are applied to the large bowel of rats, tumor growth is enhanced.

About 80–90 percent of all human cancers may be related to environmental factors, and thus, many are potentially preventable. Nutrition and diet have been suggeted to be among these environmental factors. Calorie restrictions, type and amount of dietary fat, deficiencies of certain vitamins and minerals, and dietary protein content appear to influence induction or growth of tumors in animals.

Understanding the mechanics of cancer is not simple. Many people mistakenly think cancer cells simply enter the body, mysteriously, and begin growing. Cancer cells may come from outside the body; however, many cancer cells are one's own body cells which, for some reason, have begun to grow abnormally. Cancer cells invade normal cells and interrupt normal cell activity. Out-of-control cancer cells seem to be caused by alterations to the cell that make it divide and behave abnormally. Healthy people might have abnormal cells in their bodies, but they may also have the ability to suppress development of such cells.

People who develop cancer may not have the ability to repair or destroy the abnormal cells. The effort to learn what makes cells become abnormal, keeps thousands of cancer researchers busy.

There is no way of knowing in advance if a person is susceptible to the development of cancer. For this reason, it is important that we do all we can to lower the risks of developing cancers caused by known factors. Cancer can be caused by a virus or an inherited weakness, but the majority of all cancers are caused by something people can change—their environment.

What is the connection between cancer and diet? Researchers believe cancer cells are first produced when a person is exposed to certain chemicals or conditions in the environment. The American Institute of Cancer Research states, "Certain types of diets, with their distinctive nutrient intakes, have been found either to promote or inhibit the growth of the chemically caused cancers."

Decreasing the intake of animal fats is only one factor to be considered in decreasing the risk of cancer. An increase in the consumption of fibrous foods, such as whole grains, raw fruit, and vegetables, is another. In the United States, there are from eight to fifteen times more colon cancer than in countries where unrefined foods make up most of the diet. Fiber in the diet reduces contact of cancer-producing substances in the intestinal tract and gives the body less time to absorb any cancer-causing agents. (Transit time of food through the digestive tract on a diet of unrefined foods is about 30 hours as compared to 77 hours on a diet of refined foods.) The American Institute of Cancer Research reports that foods high in vitamins A, C, E, and the mineral selenium may have a potential for cancer prevention. Foods high in vitamin A may help to lower the risk of larynx, esophagus, and lung cancer. Sources of vitamin A and carotene are dark-green and deep-yellow vegetables such as tomatoes, carrots, spinach, and fruits such as cantaloupe, apricots, and peaches. Carotene changes into vitamin A in the body. Animal studies reveal that vitamin A helps to increase the body's resistance to tumor growth. Large vitramin A supplements should be used only with the guidance of a physician.

Vegetables such as cabbage, broccoli, Brussels sprouts, and kohlrabi are also believed to help prevent cancer of the gastrointestinal and respiratory tracts.

Alcohol should be avoided. Heavy consumption of alcohol can result in liver cirrhosis, which can lead to liver cancer. Alcohol also depletes the body of some vitamins (vitamin C in particular).

Other suggestions for decreasing the risk of cancer through diet include: avoiding large quantities of coffee, avoiding artificial sweeteners unless they have been presecribed, decreasing salt-cured, salt-pickled, and smoked foods. A charcoal-broiled steak has as much benzopyrene as the smoke of 600 cigarettes. Superheating the fat of meat can form methylcholanthrene which is carcinogenic.

Foods containing unnecessary additives and quantities of artificial coloring should be avoided because some of them may cause cancer. Foods with mold or decay, such as peanuts, corn, or milk, should not be used. All fruits and vegetables should be washed thoroughly to remove residue from sprays that may have been used as pesticides.

Margaret Heckler, formerly Secretary of Health and Human Services, identifies faulty diet as the single most important cause of cancer. She states, "Too few Americans realize the simple truth that cancer is usually caused by the way they live, and its risks can be reduced by the choices they make." In spite of all that may be said in its favor, there is no "magic" food that can cure cancer. However, diet is important in the prevention of cancer. To decrease the chances of developing cancer, one should eat a diet based on the Basic Four Food Groups, keep the weight down, reduce the intake of fat, and increase the intake of fiber.

Chapter 14

Eating Out and Entertaining

The importance of restricting the intake of refined foods, visible fats, and large quantities has been stressed. How, then, does one survive eating out when he is not sure what he is ordering, or he may not know how to order the right foods in the right combination? Millions of Americans invite trouble every day by simply choosing restaurants that use large quantities of fat, for example, adding many calories to their diet.

Restaurants are big business, and when one walks into one of America's three million eating places, he could almost guess from the lavish menus offered that the number one national health problem is overweight! When dining out, one is tempted to eat more than he should. The National Restaurant Association takes pride in marketing products, and restaurants have a great responsibility when one considers that one out of every four meals is eaten away from home, not even counting those in schools, hospitals, or other institutions.

When one is watching his weight and cholesterol intake, he must give some extra thought to what he chooses to eat in a restaurant. One might eat anything he wishes if eating out is only an occasional meal, such as once a month, but when he is a frequent visitor he could have a problem, and "Dieters' specials," as advertised, may not always seem attractive. One should plan to accommodate his regular daily eating pattern, however, even in a restaurant.

For the *breakfast* meal, here are a few suggestions: modest-calorie foods like melon, grapefruit, tomato juice, or orange juice may be ordered. Usually these are listed as appetizers. However, one need not be intimidated in ordering melon or grapefruit for dessert and having juice as a beverage at any meal. A cooked cereal as opposed to a dry cereal, low-fat or non-fat milk instead of cream may be chosen. An order for bread or toast should be accompanied with a request to bring the butter in a side dish. Instead of fried eggs, one may choose poached or boiled, again cutting the fat intake. Cottage cheese as a side order complements a breakfast very well; the protein provided has less calories and less cholesterol. A pancake with a little cottage cheese and fruit, which is usually available on the breakfast menu, makes a nutritious breakfast.

Lunch also needs planning whether one eats at home or not. Salad mixtures offer opportunity for variety, and salad bars are especially inviting when one eats out. A wholesome salad may be made with garbanzos, beans, miscellaneous vegetables, and a low-calorie dressing. A soup, and a slice of bread with cheese may be added. If a dessert is desired, fruit may be chosen.

By observing these suggestions, one may have latitude for the choice of an *evening meal*. If going out to dine with friends, one should plan ahead by eating a light breakfast and a light lunch. Calories saved will allow some splurging at dinner. Care should be taken in the use of sauces, butter, gravies, and dressings. If the dessert is a big-calorie production and everyone else is having some, a small portion may be eaten and a hot beverage taken. By sipping and engaging in conversation one need not eat all the calorie-ladened dessert.

Sugar is used in abundance in desserts. The consumption of a hundred pounds of sugar each year adds up to 192,000 calories or 55 pounds of body fat to be burned off somehow. Much of the sugar consumed is hidden in fancy desserts—even to the mints at the cash register!

One should be careful to watch the size of the serving. Americans often complain about being served too much food. This complaint is usually to a friend, not the person who could do something about it. Most people would benefit if portions were relatively small. By eating large portions, many unneeded calories are added. Over a year's time the extra calories show up in extra weight. One should not hesitate to ask for small portions. One should "think lean" and stay away from visible fats.

The extra fat often used in cooking is 100 calories per tablespoon. An average-sized potato baked in its skin has only a modest 100 calories, is delicious, and can be seasoned with a smalll amount of salt, plain yogurt, or cottage cheese. It one orders mashed potatoes with added milk and butter, the calorie count is raised. French-fries are even worse offenders. Many fast foods or gourmet foods consist of battered, breaded, fried foods, which make every item high in fat and calories. Two ounces of raw onion rings provide about 18 calories compared to two ounces of French-fried onion rings that provide 166 calories. If one has a rich main dish, such as crepes or pastas, only fruit should be chosen for dessert. However, if a dessert must be eaten, then a lean entrée should be chosen preceding the dessert.

When eating out, one may still be exotic by choosing a special restaurant. Restaurants serving foods characteristic of foreign cultures often provide an excellent selection of vegetables that are not overcooked or prepared in excess fat. Spaghetti by itself, for example, is low in fat, less than one percent. But if one selects Fettucini Alfredo, rich with cream, butter, and cheese, one may then have to eat celery for a week!

Actually, food of many ethnic origins may be enjoyed if one is careful in making choices. The author is not trying to take away the fun of dining out and enjoying favorite foods or tasty new recipes. One may enjoy eating out if he does not transgress so much that he feels guilty.

The Restaurant Association is aware of increased interest in improved health through diet and exercise. The Association recently released a report, "Nutritional Expectations of Food Service Industry Patrons," which recommended modifications in life-style with particular emphasis on improved eating habits. Many restaurants are making a conscious effort to increase the variety of foods offered. An article by Jean Burkes in *Restaurant Business* states that the trends of food service are salad bars, increased use of vegetables, and the availability of salt- and sugar-free items, all signs of a growing interest of the industry in promoting sound nutrition for patrons.

So far, the discussion is about eating away from home. What if one chooses to entertain at home? An invitation to dine at one's home is the highest compliment to offer a friend. Through the centuries the greatest entertainments were always centered around dining in the home. Dinners are served in an effort to increase acquaintance with others or to celebrate special occasions. Whatever the circumstances may be, much thought and planning should go into the preparation. For example, one may take a favorite recipe and revise it by using less salt, sugar, and fat. The guests will never know the difference, and all will be better off in the long run.

Now, here are some ideas to be considered when eating out:

Appetizers

Choose

I. V-8 or tomato juice
2 Unsweetened fruit juice (small glass)
3. Clear broths or bouillon, consommé
4. Fresh vegetables
5. Sour or dill pickles
6. Fresh fruit cups

Do not choose

1. Canned fruits (contain sugar)
2. Chowders
3. Anything marinated in oil

Salads

Choose
1. Fresh fruit salad
2. Fresh vegetable salad without dressing

Do not choose
1. Salads with unknown dressings
2. Avocado

Vegetables

Choose
1. Stewed
2. Boiled
3. Steamed

Do not choose
1. Escalloped
2. Creamed
3. Au gratin
4. Fried
5. Sautéed

Potato

Choose
1. Mashed
2. Baked
3. Boiled
4. Steamed

Do not choose
1. Creamed
2. Escalloped
3. Home-fried
4. Browned
5. French-fried
6. Potato salad

Breads

Choose
1. Hard or soft rolls
2. Plain muffins
3. Biscuits
4. Crackers
5. Corn bread

Do not choose
1. Sweet rolls
2. Coffee cake
3. Danish rolls
4. Frosted rolls

Eggs

Choose
1. Soft
2. Hard
3. Poached

Do not choose
1. Scrambled
2. Fried
3. Omelet

Fats

Choose
1. Margarine
2. Salad dressing

Do not choose
1. Gravy
2. Fried foods
3. Foods with cream sauce
4. Salads with oil or dressings already mixed in

Desserts

Choose
1. Jello
2. Fresh fruit
3. Plain flavored ice cream
4. Sponge cake (leave frosting)
5. Angel food cake (leave frosting)

Do not choose
1. Custards
2. Pies
3. Sweetened canned fruits
4. Pastry

Beverages

Choose	Do not choose
1. Diet sodas	1. Cocoa
2. Coffee, decaffeinated	2. Chocolate milk (any flavored milk)
3. Tea, herb	
4. Buttermilk	3. Milk shakes
5. Whole milk	4. Regular soft drinks
6. Skim milk	5. Any beverage with unknown ingredients
7. Unsweetened fruit juices, 1 small glass, 1 fruit	

If one wishes to use the exchange list, the following suggestions may be helpful:

Exchanges for Special Dishes

Special Dish	Amount	Food Exchanges
Beef stew	1 cup	2 protein 1 bread 2 fat
Baked beans and frankfurters	2	3 protein
Baked Beans	4 rounded tablespoons	2 breads
Baked macaroni and cheese	1 cup	1 milk 1 protein 2 bread
Corned beef hash, canned	¾ cup	3 protein 1 bread
Coleslaw	½ cup	1 vegetable (Group A) 1 fat
Italian spaghetti	1 serving (1 cup spaghetti) 2 small meat balls ½ cup sauce	2 ½ bread 3 protein 2 fat
Chop suey (chicken)	1 cup	1 bread 1 protein
Pancakes	2 pancakes (4" diameter)	1 bread 1 fat
French-fried potatoes	5 pieces, 2" × ½" × ½"	1 bread 1 fat
Potato chips	15 medium (2" diameter) 10 large (3" diameter)	1 bread or 2 fat
Poultry with stuffing	4 ounces poultry ⅓ cup stuffing	4 protein 1 bread 1 fat
Chili con carne with beans	1 cup	2 bread 2 protein

Chapter 15

Your Money's Worth in Foods

With the cost of living today, who isn't concerned about the dollars required for food? Following are suggestions to help reduce those food bills, and, at the same time, provide guidance so that one may be well nourished for less money.

There are no simple dollars-and-cents answers to the question of food purchases; however, guidelines may be helpful in controlling cost while spending enough to provide the family with an adequate diet.

There are many combinations of foods at various levels of cost that will provide the nutrients for a well-balanced diet. Three basic food plans will help in determining how much one might reasonably spend—low cost, moderate cost, and liberal cost. Each cost reflects buying practices of low, middle, and high income families. The lower the cost, the more time, interest, and skill required to plan, buy, and prepare foods.

Any pattern that suits the family is all right if the pattern does two things: 1) provides for regular meals, including a nutritious breakfast; and 2) allows for a variety of foods—the Basic Four Food Groups.

The family savings begin at home, before one goes to the market, by making a tentative menu plan for the next few days or for a week. Then the shopping list should be prepared. Shopping is a challenge, but here are a few basic ideas:

1. Make careful and complete lists.
2. Take only enough money as allowed in the budget.
3. Write no checks, to avoid being tempted to spend more money than planned.
4. Shop only once a week.
5. Don't yield to temptation or impulse buying.
6. Forget "convenience foods"—the price is more than other foods.
7. Watch for specials—don't stock up needlessly.
8. Compare frozen, fresh, and canned—then select the best bargain.

9. Read all labels for nutritional contents.
10. Check unit prices.
11. Save coupons—use them when appropriate.
12. Trade coupons with friends.
13. Shop in at least two stores for best bargains.
14. Buy smaller sizes—cost is less; for example, apples.
15. Look down and bend down at supermarkets—more expensive items are on upper shelves.

One needs to consider what quantity of each item to buy. Usually foods in large containers cost less per unit weight than in small containers, but if food is left over and eventually thrown out, the buy is not considered wise. If using leftovers means monotonous meals, and the food cannot be stored properly and conveniently, the purchasing plan should be revised. The following should be considered:

1. Check prices in different stores for foods bought regularly.
2. Decide which store offers reasonable prices and features that are important, such as variety, quality foods, off-street parking.
3. Choose a large independent store for:
   a. Variety,
   b. Shopping convenience,
   c. Lower prices.

For certain foods, one might prefer a specialty shop, such as a bakery or vegetable stand, because the quality may be higher or the price lower.

Usually efficiency dictates choosing a convenient, reasonably-priced store and staying with it. Store hopping for an advertised special usually costs more because of wasted time and increased wear-and-tear in transportation.

When is the best time to shop? When the store is not crowded and one is not hurried and pushed about. Time will enable one to read the labels, compare prices, and get acquainted with new food products. One should give food purchasing the attention it deserves.

Other ways to cut costs include:

1. Be able to substitute one vegetable or fruit for another.
2. Learn to spot real quality, not just "good looking produce."
3. Limit purchases of perishable foods to the amounts that can be used while they are still fresh.
4. Take advantage of seasonal abundance.
5. Watch for specials on canned and frozen products the family likes.
6. Try lower-priced brands.
7. Check for grades on canned products—color, texture, flavor, shape, uniformity of size, and freedom from defects.
8. Make sauces for vegetables.
9. Choose cooked cereals—the cost is lower.
10. Save on day-old bread and other baked goods.
11. Buy fresh milk from the store. Home-delivered milk costs more.
12. Buy ½ or gallon containers if possible, to use without waste.
13. Use evaporated or non-fat milk in cooking.
14. Choose natural cheeses—they cost less than processed cheeses.

15. Try to shop alone so attention is not diverted.
16. Shop days when the foods are freshest and most plentiful, usually toward the end of the week.
17. Eat before shopping so you are less likely to make unnecessary purchases because of hunger.

Using these guidelines, one saves dollars, improves eating, and thus contributes to health and happiness!

A caution to remember: a "bargain" is not a bargain unless the item can be used. Sometimes one is tempted to buy when the item is really not needed. Avoid unnecessary stockpiling. A "bargain" may not be a bargain even though the price may be reduced!

Chapter 16

Learning to Cope with Stress

For some people, stress is chronic and endless, seemingly the primary force of their personalities. Such aggressive, hard-driving personalities may be headed for trouble.

Stress is the reaction of the body to any event which requires the adjustment of body "machinery" to meet a crisis or emergency. Stress is caused by pressure, strain, urgency, intense effort necessary to meet assignments and goals. Just the wear-and-tear of living in today's world can be stressful. Everything one does is involved with stress—even love or hate. Dr. Hans Selye observed that the absence of harmful stress depends largely upon feelings of gratitude and goodwill; its presence depends on their negative counterpart, hatred, with the urge for revenge. Stress is an everyday fact of life; one cannot avoid stress. The physical exertion of work or play is a type of stress, but actually beneficial for people. What makes or breaks one is not stress itself but the ability or inability to handle stressful situations. Stress may have different effects on different people.

From the time one gets up in the morning until retirement at night, there are often pressures of one kind or another. Getting dressed in haste and ready for work, often eating on the run, rushing to catch a bus or meet someone, even driving and at the same time indulging in such activity as combing hair, putting on makeup, drinking a cup of coffee while watching signals, dodging traffic, and making one last leap to get to the desk on time—in all such circumstances people create a lot of their own stress and anxiety.

Much anxiety could be avoided by planning—allowing time for necessary preparations so that one arrives promptly at the chosen destination. Because many live in the "fast lane," feeling constantly pressured, the chances are their eating habits—not to mention the nutritional adequacy of their diets—should be of some concern.

One experiences stress from three basic sources: one's environment, one's body, and one's thoughts, and various types of stress in varying degrees are encountered in everyday living such as physical, mental, and emotional stress. The stress caused by certain experiences may even weaken the body's resistance, increasing its susceptibility to diseases or involvement with accidents. Sometimes, however, stress may be advantageous. Learning to balance mental exertion with manual labor is often all that is needed.

One's ability to manage stress is governed by three factors: 1) the number of stressful situations; 2) the personality which determines how one reacts to situations; and 3) the life-style as it affects the capacity of the body to resist stress. One can change all these factors if he chooses to manage stress before stress manages him. Making an effort to restructure activities in order to be able to cope with problems will go a long way in producing a happy, healthy life.

One of the first steps in controlling stress is to identify those situations that cause or contribute to the "uptight condition."

The author shares what has worked for her for over thirty years. By nature, she is an early riser, so "up and at it" is her motto. Getting up at an early hour, reading something devotional, something inspirational, something that will contribute to the stamina needed for the day is the first priority. After personal preparations are made for the day, an adequate breakfast is the next priority, a meal consisting of a hot, whole-grain cereal, fruit, and an egg or tofu. If there is any time, a few household duties may be done, but not at the expense of being late for work or not being ready for the assignments of the day.

One should make a conscious effort to slow down, to take a few minutes to analyze himself and the problems contributing to the stress. A few questions to ask are: "Am I ambitious, competitive, always punctual, feeling behind in work, always worrying about deadlines, annoyed with delays in traffic, impatient in conversation, talking and eating rapidly, trying to do two things at once?"

Each person has the power to control much of what goes on in his life. But he must make a plan and follow it in order to be able to handle the unexpected. One's mental attitude is vitally important. Adequate nutrition, rest, and exercise, keeping physically fit, will help in handling any task.

There are also pleasurable situations involving stress and tension—these can be exhilarating. But the stress that nags, causes intense and persistent fear, anger, frustration, and worry threatens one's well-being. If not properly handled, this type of stress can break down a person physically. The buildup of stress without release of tension leads to trouble. Where there is a steady strain, one may experience a variety of symptoms such as irritability, frequent headaches, or digestive distress. These are signals indicating that a change needs to be made. Strong emotions cause bodily changes because emotions are meant to make one act. When a person feels helpless or unable to cope with a situation, he is in a vulnerable position that may contribute to various problems, including disease.

Some of the most common illnesses caused in various degrees by stress include acne and skin disorders, alcoholism, allergies, arthritis, asthma, colitis, constipation, diarrhea, gout, headaches, heart disease, hypertension, nervous breakdowns, ulcers. Of course, some people are more adversely affected by stress than others.

One's disposition, attitudes, and circumstances, all help to "make or break." If a person is competitive, impatient, and time-oriented, then being successful and making things happen are very important. One tends to look to success and possessions to have a feeling of well-being and acceptance. If, on the other hand, a person is easy-going, he seldom becomes impatient or worried about time; rather, he tends to make decisions, and not to be unduly influenced by the opinions of others.

One may ask what can be done to counteract and relieve stress. The first requisite is to learn to relax—to find a quiet place for relaxing, resting, reading, or just doing something that one enjoys. Relaxing in a hot tub, having someone gently massage tense neck or back muscles, talking with a close friend may suffice. Happiness is a choice, and every day one should choose to do that which will bring the most happiness to himself and to others—choose to do worthwhile activities that will bring a sense of self-worth.

Projects and activities such as painting, sewing, writing, hiking, carpentry, photography may also help one to relax. The activity chosen should bring pleasure, release—and relaxation. Activities with close friends can often be satisfying.

Exercise is an activity that promotes relaxation. There are many exercises that lessen stress, relieve frustration and boredom, release aggressive feelings, as well as help to control weight. Exercise gives a person a feeling of well-being, self-confidence, and accomplishment. Exercise gives a surge of energy as well as a happy outlook. Even simple breathing exercises can help one relax, or just breathing properly, wearing loose clothing, and being comfortable.

The kind of exercise one chooses depends on his present condition of health and on what he enjoys doing. Before undertaking strenuous exercise, the advice of a physician should be obtained. Walking is a simple, safe exercise for almost anyone, at any age. One can go at the pace that is best suited for him, doing what is a pleasure, not a chore.

Taking a minute to stretch helps relieve body tension. If a person feels tension in the back of the neck and shoulder area, he may rotate the head slowly in one direction, then in the opposite direction, or he may stretch the arms, torso, and legs. There are sample exercises from which one may choose. Whatever exercise one selects to do, should be done every day to bring satisfaction. Breathing is essential for life and energy. Proper breathing habits may be an antidote to stress.

In addition to relaxation and exercise, a third way to handle stress is to eat wisely. When one is under stress, the nutritional needs increase, the body uses food more rapidly; hence, careful attention should be given to providing the body with the right nutrients. The body needs nutrients to repair the damage caused by stress. Stress puts pressure on the nerves.

Healthy nerves need vitamin B complex. If there is a deficiency, tiredness and general lowering of health will be noticed. The best source for B complex vitamins is whole-grain cereals, egg yolk, milk, most vegetables, especially peas and beans. Since the B vitamins are water soluble, the foods providing these vitamins should be cooked in a minimum of water to avoid loss of nutrients. Enzymes also contribute to the release of nutrients during digestion. Calcium can be assimilated only if vitamin D is present. Therefore, one should increase the calcium foods by eating milk, eggs, cheese, green-leafy and yellow vegetables, foods high in the B vitamins. One should reduce the intake of refined sweets because these "use up" available vitamin B. Some time spent outdoors in the sunshine is an excellent way to obtain vitamin D.

Foods high in iron should be eaten for the formation of hemoglobin which carries oxygen to the cells. A well-balanced diet should be eaten—one that includes proteins, carbohydrates, fats, vitamins, and minerals. The Basic Four Food Groups should be the basis of the everyday diet, including fresh fruits and vegetables; cereals, grains, eggs, nuts, legumes, and other sources of proteins; and dairy products.

Eating patterns that provide low-fat, low-sugar, and low-salt intake are important in providing adequate nutrition, and also in watching one's weight. Excess weight puts extra strain on the body. Weight constricts the heart muscles and arteries, hampers respiration and digestion, and makes the body work much harder than it should. One ought to stay within 10 pounds of ideal weight. Stress often affects the quantity one eats, triggering a desire to overeat.

Each person holds the key to improved health and quality of life if he learns to handle stress, if he learns to cope with physical and/or mental strain. When one fails to plan adequately, one usually does not attain the desired goals, and stress is bound to occur.

Simple guidelines for coping with stress include:

1. Be alert to the body's physical reactions to stress (headaches, stomach churning, clammy hands).
2. Ask, "Am I taking on too much?"
3. Balance work with play.
4. Learn to loaf a bit, "get away from it all," pick a hobby.
5. Get enough sleep and rest.
6. Work off tensions by some physical function.

7. Talk about problems with close friends.
8. Learn to accept what cannot be changed.
9. Make time an ally, not a master.
10. Avoid self-medication.
11. Don't let things drift.
12. Try to avoid as much worry as possible.
13. If the job is a problem, consider changing position and/or locale.
14. Arrange for privacy.
15. Don't blame others.
16. Develop positive attitudes toward the source of stress-producing pressures.
17. Exercise options wherever possible, and don't insist on winning.
18. Take a few minutes out of each day just for one's self.
19. Capitalize on areas of independent, creative responsibility.
20. Choose to incorporate into your life alternatives to the many individual sources of anxiety, confusion, and unnecessary stimulation.
21. Look beyond immediate and temporary problems, study long-term perspectives in relation to problem-solving.
22. Keep your work and non-work life as separate as possible.

Someone has said, laugh and live longer. The Good Book also has wise counsel: "A merry heart doeth good like a medicine." One should not be afraid to tell a joke, be funny, and above all have a sense of humor. And—eternal optimism is the key to overcoming some of the problems that confront everyone every day.

One needs to learn to play a bit, to get away from it all, to take a vacation, to read an interesting book, to have some fun every day, and not to take himself or details too seriously. The biggest business in which any person may invest and which will bring the greatest profit is his health. Each person needs to make the most of the state of health that he has now. These simple suggestions, if followed, will surely result in improved physical and mental health.

The practice of positive thinking goes a long way in the treatment of either a real or unreal situation. One can train himself to cope with stress by relaxing away anxiety and stress reactions. Learning to relax efficiently is the foundation stone for coping with stress.

Learning to have a happy, loving, positive attitude will contribute to the quality of life. The reader has the power within himself to learn successful ways to cope with stress.

Stress often makes people more vulnerable to illness. When a person understands why he gets sick, then he/she may be able to do something about the situations which are the causes.

Everybody has some stress. In fact, stress just goes with being human. But too much stress and, surprisingly, too little stress, cause difficulty and can lead to *distress*.

Stress and the human being may be compared to tension on a violin string. The string has to be taut to produce a healthy sound. If the string is limp, there will be no music. But if the string is too "tight," it could snap. So, somewhere in-between seems to be best.

Each person has his/her own stress-tolerance level—the level at which he/she feels most comfortable and productive. Too little stress makes for a boring life. Too much stress makes him/her more vulnerable to illness

Chapter 17

Managing Depression

Depression may be caused by many circumstances. These include love, grief, ill health, social rejection, loneliness, unhappiness, finance, attitudes, marriage, divorce—to name a few that may affect how one meets life each day. The mind is constantly under stress from the outside (the environment and people) and from within (emotional reactions). Conflicts are unavoidable; some are resolved without too much strain, while others may be complex. When conflicts are evaded, the mind and body suffer damage. Political problems, economic problems, illnesses may trigger depression. Some people live in a withering, negative world.

The author has always been an optimist, living with a positive attitude, but effort and thought must be exercised in order to avoid depression. Attitude has much to do with the way one handles problems. Thinking positively and combining all one's efforts in one direction may be helpful. Being thankful for all the blessings which most people are prone to take for granted contributes to strengthening the positive attitude. Maintaining a cheerful disposition and working with a strong will can bring fulfillment to one's needs and goals. Some people give up too easily.

A friend's formula for success has been used many times in helping others, and the author would like to share it with the reader. The author had just hired a person to fill a "not-so-easy" position. Knowing that the friend would meet opposition and problems, a plan was devised. The friend's attitude was unusual in that she was bound to succeed, and she did. But as the position was discussed and its problems were reviewed, she thought a second, and said emphatically, "Nothing comes easy, but I will *make* it happen." "I will make it happen" reflects an important attitude in meeting life's goals and ambitions.

Depression comes from a variety of causes or circumstances. Illness is often a reason for depression. Loneliness is a contributing factor. A friend of the author was prone to depression and would often cry for long periods of time. As the situation was discussed, the author soon discovered the reason this person was depressed. If the sky was cloudy, dark, or rainy, she was depressed. She explained that she had a friend that felt the same way. Whenever the sky was dark, her friend would pull the shades and turn on the lights. By listening for a short time, the truth was revealed. This person did not try to meet depression, she just *provided for it*. Everyone has problems, loneliness, illness, but not everyone allows himself to become depressed.

Losses and grief are not easy to deal with. To talk about the loss with a close friend, letting the tears flow, and not repressing the feeling may be a way of saying "goodbye" to the lost person or object.

Jerome Marmorstein, M.D. in *The Psychometabolic Blues*, discusses "Mourning and Depression" in this manner:

"When a family member is lost through death, the immediate reaction is often guilt over what could have been done to foresee and prevent it. This guilt occurs whether or not there is any personal responsibility involved. Differentiating the depression that occurs as a part of normal mourning from that which is clinically abnormal cannot usually be determined immediately after the death of a family member. The intensity of the sadness and the occurrence of psychosomatic symptoms such as loss of appetite and insomnia are identical. At times, feelings of guilt may seem more intense in those who will go on to develop the more prolonged abnormal depression. In every sense, mourning is a period of intense depression. But its duration is limited to an appropriate period for the particular circumstance. Usually, this is up to several months for the major symptoms, with lesser degrees of depression lasting for one or two years. If the duration of the intense period of depression persists more than a few months, with continuing severe psychosomatic symptoms, then one might be experiencing a true clinical depression and should seek benefit from professional help. Otherwise, the depression might persist for years. Even for normal mourning, it is often helpful to see one's personal physician for whatever support he could offer.

"The quality of the relationship before death can be a great influence. Paradoxically, we have observed that the death of a spouse in a happy marriage may be less likely to cause prolonged depression than in an unhappy marriage. Also, a surviving son or daughter is less likely to experience prolonged depression if there was a comfortable relationship with the parent. These observations might be explained by the amount of guilt generated by regrets over unresolved conflicts. Unselfish love may be the capacity to let go of a loved one if it should be necessary.

"The immediate circumstances surrounding the death of a family member will also influence the amount of guilt generated. It may seem obvious that a suicide involving marital conflict may generate more guilt than death from natural causes. What may not be obvious is that the suicide and the marital stress may have had the same underlying cause—depression in the one who committed suicide. Often this is related primarily to factors outside of the marriage, and the surviving spouse assumes a burden of guilt that is not deserved. Even when a spouse dies of natural causes, the survivor often feels that he or she should have sought medical help sooner, or somehow foreseen the problem.

"Another important circumstance is whether the survivor has had an opportunity to prepare for the death of the loved one. Sudden, unexpected death, without a preceding period of illness, may not allow the psychological preparation afforded by a chronic illness. The disbelief and denial that often follows prevents the usual expression of grief and may predispose one to the development of a delayed onset of depression." *

Depression must be shunned—avoided! An activity should be chosen that will occupy the time and mind so that if depression is a problem, some provision is made to avoid being overcome. People should be thankful for the pluses in their environment and foster a few close, supportive friends who will be happy to help bridge difficult periods of life.

Intelligent eating habits contribute significantly to well-being and a healthy mental attitude. Nutrition has become a concern of the Nation especially since people have become aware that this country is not a nutritionally well-fed Nation. Many poor choices in people's eating habits result in malnutrition. Could there be any correlation between a malnourished body and a malnourished mind? The brain is a very important organ in governing the functions of the body.

When malnutrition is present, the brain does not function as well. The brain is closely connected with the stomach, and brain power has so often been drawn upon to aid weakened digestive organs that the brain itself becomes weakened, depressed, congested. Although humanity's most precious possession is the human brain, one has only the slightest idea of how it works.

A person's habits should be brought under the control of the mind. Mental and moral power are dependent upon physical health. There is an intimate relation between the mind and the body, and, in order to reach a standard of moral and intellectual attainment, the controls that guide the physical being must be heeded.

Day-to-day dispositions and attitudes are largely controlled by what is eaten. For instance, if one overeats, the physical organs are taxed and the brain beclouded. On the other hand, if nutritious meals are eaten and the principles of health followed, a person's outlook on life becomes vastly different.

The emotions many times dictate when and what should be eaten. Tests over the years reveal the extent to which people allow circumstances and conditions to control their actions.

Here are a few questions one may ask:

1. Do I eat excessively when bored or depressed?
2. Do I eat foods that I know are not good for me?
3. Do I prefer eating alone?
4. Do I feel conspicuous when eating with others?
5. Do I fear weight gain?
6. Do I eat or drink in secrecy?
7. Do I gulp my food?
8. Do I have eating binges?
9. Do I stuff myself?
10. Do I have waves of anger or hostility?

The author suggests that if one is ill, he should seek professional help and follow the doctor's advice. However, visualizing being well and thinking about what one will do when the conditions change, reading an interesting book or a funny article or story, having an attitude of happiness, thankfulness, and even daring to laugh a bit—these attitudes and activities can foster a healthy mental attitude. All one has to do is to look about and see that other people have problems also; realizing that one's condition could be worse goes a long way toward changing attitude. Thinking strong, giving cheer and courage to others, trying to be a happy person are conducive to handling difficulties. People need to get in touch with themselves and make necessary changes in their mental attitude. Thinking well of one's self contributes to total health. A healthy mind influences a healthy body.

One should not allow depression to rule. Everyone has something to be thankful for, and something worthwhile to think about. Each person should be aware of his potential. Thinking positively, setting goals, and attempting to change one's self-image are acts of accomplishment that are important for the "whole" person.

Psychologists help people to overcome depression by teaching them how to increase their rewarding activities and to learn a more positive way of thinking about themselves. Studies of depressed people have shown that they experience a low rate of rewarding events and a high rate of adverse events. One theory of depression is that depressed people act in ways which reduce the amount of positive interactions they have with the world, especially with other people. This reduction may result in increasing the depression. Another theory of depression is that depressed people have a negative view of themselves, the world, and the future; such a view may cause them to interpret events in negative ways and, thus, to feel depressed. This negative view is caused by errors of thinking which the depressed person may filter or distort so that he actually clings to painful attitudes despite objective evidence to the contrary. Both theoretical positions advocate similar treatments which have been found to be effective in relieving depression. These treatments involve increasing pleasant events, learning social skills (e.g., assertiveness) which lead to more positive and less adverse social experiences, and learning to interpret events in positive ways.

Having a positive mental attitude does not magically make things turn out well. However, such an attitude enables one to find joy in living and to face problems in a manner which is healthy and adaptive both mentally and physically. A positive mental attitude enables one to be at his best and to be sensitive and aware of the possibilities for good, for health, for growth, and for wholeness in the situations that are encountered in daily living. A positive mental attitude does not deny or distort reality. Rather, it sees below the surface of reality and facilitates whatever potential for good that can be realized. In the face of evil or pain, a positive mental attitude is not characterized by negative optimism or happiness but by re-demptiveness, forgiveness, and healing. Some might say that the healing powers of a positive mental attitude are only a mental "trick" that people play on themselves. If so, then food and drink are physical "tricks" as well, for a positive attitude provides nourishment, energy, and strength. To be worthwhile, a positive mental attitude does not have to enable one to overcome all adversities, but only to deal with them as well as possible so that suffering is lessened, if not completely relieved, and opportunities for joy are not overlooked.

*From *The Psychometabolic Blues.* Copyright ©1979 by Jerome Marmorstein and Nanette Marmorstein. Used by permission of Woodbridge Press, Santa Barbara, CA 93160.

Chapter 18
Reaching Your Goal

In the preceding chapters preventive maintenance and total health have been stressed. Ways of avoiding illness are important to know. Human beings can replace machinery, but how can damaged, worn-out body parts be replaced? To neglect the body is expensive business. Health, happiness, and energy cannot be purchased with money. These are values that must be acquired from a practice of right principles.

Today the whole world embraces the idea of the need for adequate nutrition. If the reader has taken the advice in the preceding chapters seriously, he should be thinking about setting realistic goals that will assist him in making changes in his life-style. To drift aimlessly is fatal; he must steer his course. To structure a goal is like having a road map to guide over the route. Once the skill is acquired, a habit is formed. Well-established habits are essential to maintaining health.

The potential for ultimate health derives from utilizing information and capacities which exist, but which if unused avail nothing. Realizing one's potential involves experiencing life at its fullest, and realizing that one is alive and has a firm lease on life.

Everyone can be in charge of his life and make wise choices to remove self-imposed obstacles that might limit the degree of preventive maintenance in health.

What are some of the changes that need to be considered? To recapitulate: there is a growing awareness of the importance in cutting back on the amount of sugar used, of decreasing the amount of salt used, of increasing the amount of fibrous food eaten, and considering carefully the quality and quantity of fat consumed. One should realize the importance of balancing the food intake with the energy needs for the day. Learning how to eat less and be satisfied can be accomplished only with an attitude that is willing and ready for change. Leaving the table a bit hungry is wise. When one can exercise this kind of concern and control, he is in charge—he is being positive.

Exercise is an integral component in formulating worthwhile goals. One needs to choose the appropriate changes to be made in his life-style with a plan as to how these changes may be achieved. *Goals* are where the action is. Goals give meaning and purpose, and enhance achievement.

One needs to consider increasing the fruits and vegetables eaten each day. These contain many nutrients, a large amount of fiber, and are very low in calories. Fruits and vegetables also contain a large amount of moisture. These foods are most healthful, contain natural sugars, and do not raise blood cholesterol levels. The carbohydrate level of some fruits is more than others. For example, grapes, 1 cup = 106 calories; watermelon, 1 cup = 52 calories. There are many healthful, low-calorie snacks, such as popcorn without butter, fruits, and vegetables.

With additional information and improved health habits, one is better equipped to face each day. One can kill himself by being negligent and careless, but by careful, preventive maintenance, one may not only have a longer life, but be in a position to enjoy the *quality* of a longer life. This volume presents a new discipline for acquiring adequate nutrition as it is related to the needs of all ages from all walks of life.

The ability to structure properly changes in life-style and to set goals is essential to realizing one's potential. A fascinating aspect of goal-setting is the benefits that accrue to those who have a purpose in living.

There is a marked relationship between the standards of one's friends and one's goal-setting. Family support is often needed to succeed. Many times setting a sub-goal is a preferred plan. When the sub-goal is reached, achieving the total goal may be relatively easy. Each one controls the magnitude of the risks he chooses to accept in reaching a desired goal.

By making a plan for whatever changes are desired, the chances to succeed are a thousand times better. Writing out what is desired in health, happiness, friends, success, or honor may be advantageous. The first step toward achievement is to make up one's mind, then pursue the decision diligently. Courage, hope, faith, sympathy, and love promote health and prolong life. A peaceful mind, a cheerful spirit assure health to the body and strength to the soul.

A question one may ask is, "Do my daily health habits reveal an awareness of the link between health of body and health of mind?" None knows exactly what his fate might have been had he lived differently. The relationship between the mind and the body is re-markably intimate.

In the previous chapters there has been a discussion of many principles, of certain concepts that may be new, an invasion of unfamiliar territories, a discovery of improved ways resulting from possible changes in life-style. As one endeavors to apply these ideas in his personal life, one should be strengthened in determination to meet the needs of the body on a day-to-day basis. There will always be problems to solve, circumstances to change, and stresses with which to cope. A well-nourished body will help greatly in meeting the needs of each day.

The reader is invited to undertake an adventure in health by utilizing the information here presented to insure a full and happy life. In other words, *Put Life Into Living!*

Section II: Recipes

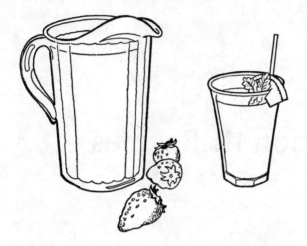

Beverages

Banana-Pineapple Drink

1 46-ounce can unsweetened
  pineapple juice (cool)
4 bananas

1. Mix above ingredients.
2. Whiz in blender and serve.

Yield: 6 8-ounce servings.

Carbohydrate, 50.0 grams; Protein, 1.8 grams; Fat, 0.3 gram.
Calories, 210 per serving.

Note: For a variation, add 15 unsweetened frozen strawberries.

Golden Punch

2 cups buttermilk   Orange rind as desired
1½ cups orange juice   2 teaspoons sugar (optional)

1. Beat or shake all ingredients together so that the mixture is
   smooth and frothy.
2. Chill and serve.

Yield: 4 servings; *serving:* 1 cup.

Carbohydrate, 16.5 grams; Protein, 4.4 grams; Fat, .1 gram.
Calories, 85 per serving.

Orange-Banana Punch

3 medium bananas, mashed   3 cups orange juice
½ cup non-fat milk powder

1. Blend mashed bananas with dry milk powder.
2. Blend in orange juice and beat until light and fluffy.
3. Chill and serve.

Yield: 4 cups; *serving:* 1 cup.

Carbohydrate, 54 grams; Protein, 4 grams; Fat, .8 gram.
Calories, 239 per serving.

Lime Sherbet Punch

2 liter bottles of 7-UP
2½ pounds lime sherbet

1. Pour 7-UP in bowl.
2. Scoop sherbet into the bowl.
3. Stir and serve.

Yield: 20 servings; *serving:* 6.7 ounces

Carbohydrate, 31.0 grams; Protein, .4 gram; Fat, .7 gram.
Calories, 130 per serving.

Note: Orange or raspberry sherbet may be used instead of lime.

Strawberry Punch

3 small packages   2 bananas
  strawberries, frozen   Water to make 1 gallon
¾ cup strawberry syrup
1 6-ounce can lemonade

1. Put frozen strawberries in blender.
2. Add strawberry syrup, lemonade, and bananas.
3. Blend together.
4. Remove and put in gallon container.
5. Add enough water and/or ice to make 1 gallon.
6. Mix well.

Yield: 1 gallon.

Carbohydrate, 47.5 grams; Protein, 3.2 grams; Fat, 1.8 grams.
Calories, 219 per 8-ounce serving.

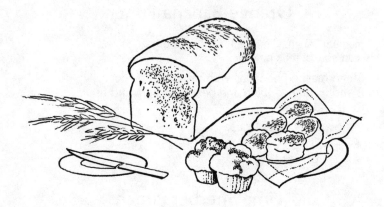

Whole Grains in Breads

Food is a universal language, a necessity for life—and *bread* is a common denominator of all cultures. Bread, in a wealth of varieties, is basic. Since about ten percent of the total intake of nutrients per day is derived from bread, the preparation of delicious, nutritious bread is of fundamental importance.

Some breads are made with yeast, and some are "quick breads." However, using active, dry yeast makes breadmaking easy. Best of all, the yeast helps to make bread one of the most enjoyable and creative of all cooking arts.

The methods described in this chapter involve bread-making by hand. Undoubtedly, everyone has eaten well-prepared bread and poorly prepared bread. There are certain basic steps for good bread-making. First, the essentials: freshness and quality of the flours top the list. Hard, spring wheat flour is best for breadmaking, with its high gluten content. A mixture of flours increases the bread's nutritive value because the nutrients of one flour supplement those of the others. The flours should be at room temperature (though stored in a cool place). Once breadmaking has commenced, the temperature must be kept constant. If, in the mixing and rising of bread, the dough becomes too warm, an off-flavor will develop. If the temperature is too cool, the rising process is prolonged.

The yeast plant grows best at a temperature of 84 degrees. The yeast should be dissolved in a small amount of liquid according to the directions. Salt and fat retard the growth of the yeast and should not be added to a yeast mixture until it has grown strongly and become lively by feeding on sugar and starch. Too much sugar will also retard the action of the yeast.

Whole-Wheat Bread Recipe

½ cup warm water
1 package dry yeast

Combine and let stand for 10 minutes.

2 cups warm water	1 tablespoon oil
½ tablespoon salt	½ cup wheat germ
¼ cup brewers' yeast	2 cups whole-wheat flour
½ cup molasses	3½ cups unbleached white flour
1 tablespoon brown sugar	

Mix together the remaining ingredients with about half of the flour, then add the yeast mixture and mix until smooth. If a mixture of flours is being added, develop the gluten of the wheat flour in the batter by beating with a sturdy spoon thoroughly before adding the other flours. Continue adding the remaining flour as required to make the dough stiff enough to knead by hand. Some wheats absorb more liquid than others.

The kneading procedure is highly important in breadmaking. Flour the hands,then turn out the dough onto a floured breadboard and knead by folding the dough over forward and pushing it down and away with the heel of the hand in a quick rocking motion; turn dough a quarter turn, and repeat until the dough is smooth and elastic and does not stick to the board. A poor job of kneading the dough before the first rising period cannot be remedied. About 200 strokes or five to seven minutes of kneading are necessary to form a smooth dough.

Now it is time to prepare the dough and climate for the rising process. Press the dough into a lightly oiled bowl large enough to allow for the rising. Then turn the dough over so that the surface of the dough is greased and will stretch easily as it rises. Cover the dough with wax paper and a towel. Let it rise in a warm place (80–85°).

Allow the dough to rise until it is double in bulk (2 to 2½ hours if the dough is kept at 80°F). When the dough has risen enough, punch it down by plunging the fist into the center of the dough, then fold the edges to the center. Turn the dough upside down in the bowl, and cover. Let the dough rise again in a warm place until it doubles in bulk—about 45 minutes. When the dough is ready to mold into loaves, punch it down and divide into sections depending on the number of loaves to be made. Flatten the dough evenly into oblong shape, pressing out the air. Shape the dough into loaves by rolling it up tightly and pressing the edges to seal. Turn the ends under and tuck in so the edges touch the sides of the pan snugly and smoothly.

Never fill the pans too full. Give plenty of room for expansion without having to billow over the sides of the pans, causing cracked-open, browned crusts. Place in oiled loaf pan, seam side down. Oil the top of the loaf and cover. Let the loaf rise until the sides reach the top of the pan and the center is well-rounded.

The oven should be preheated before the bread is ready to be baked. A wise idea is to turn the oven on when molding the loaves so the kitchen is warm and helps the bread to rise quickly. Do not allow the bread to overrise. Test the loaf by touching gently at a corner. If a slight indentation remains, the loaf is ready for baking.

For baking, place the loaf pans gently in the hot oven (about 375°F), avoiding contact with each other or the sides of the oven. Bake the loaves until a deep, golden brown is apparent. To test the loaf, tap the crust, which should sound hollow when the loaf is done. The loaves should be small and thoroughly baked. No odor of yeast should be present in the bread when the loaf is taken out.

Remove the loaves from the pans. Place the loaves on wire cooling racks away from drafts. Lightly brushing the crust of each loaf with hot water immediately after taking from the pans will insure a tender crust. Do not cover baked bread while it is cooling.

Once a person is familiar with the process of baking bread, the imagination may have free rein in experimenting with different ingredients and combinations. For example, the use of multiple whole grains will be highly rewarding. Bread freezes well, so several kinds may be prepared at one time and kept in the freezer.

Bread is one of man's oldest foods, and people continue to recognize its value in the diet. Today's homemaker can turn out a delicious loaf of bread, a sure way to make the family happy. The recipes that are suggested are nutritious, tasty, and full of natural nutrients. (If at all possible, use fresh, hard wheats, and grind the flour just before each baking to avoid loss of nutrients and to insure flavorful bread.)

All-Bran Muffins

¾ cup milk
1 cup bran (All-Bran, Bran Buds, Bran Shreds)
1 cup flour
1 tablespoon baking powder

3 tablespoons sugar
¼ teaspoon salt
1 egg, well-beaten
3 tablespoons margarine, melted

1. Pour milk over bran in mixing bowl.
2. Sift together dry ingredients. Add egg and margarine to bran mixture.
3. Add dry ingredients, mixing as little as possible.
4. Bake in well-oiled muffin pan at 425°F for 25 minutes.
5. Honey Glaze may be added if desired. See following recipe for Honey Glaze.

Yield: 10–12 muffins; serving: 1 muffin.

Carbohydrate, 31.0 grams; Protein, 4.7 grams; Fat, 7.0 grams. Calories, 206 per muffin.

Honey Glaze

¼ cup honey
1 cup water
1 cup sugar, granulated

1 cup brown sugar
¾ cup shortening
1 cup pecans, chopped

1. Combine all ingredients except pecans, and mix until smooth.
2. In each muffin tin cup place some pecans, some Honey Glaze, and some batter.
3. Bake as directed.

Muffin with Honey Glaze:

Carbohydrate, 39.0 grams; Protein, 5.0 grams; Fat, 12.0 grams.
Calories, 284 per muffin.

Corn Bread

1⅔ cups cornmeal
⅓ cup unbleached white or whole-wheat flour
¼ cup sugar
1 teaspoon salt

2 teaspoons baking powder
2 cups skim milk
¼ cup corn oil
2 eggs

1. Combine cornmeal, flour, sugar, salt, and baking powder; mix together.
2. Add milk, oil, and eggs. Mix until smooth.
3. Pour batter ½ inch deep into greased cake pan. The shallow amount of batter will yield a thin and crisp corn bread.
4. Bake in a 400°F oven for 20 minutes or until batter is firm to the touch and lightly browned.
5. Cut into squares and serve at once.

Yield: 10 servings.

Carbohydrate, 30.6 grams; Protein, 5.7 grams; Fat, 7.9 grams.
Calories, 216 per serving.

Cheddar-Bran Muffins

1¼ cups buttermilk
1 cup whole bran
2 tablespoons oil
3 tablespoons sugar
1 egg

1½ cups sifted all-purpose flour
1½ teaspoons baking powder
½ teaspoon soda
½ cup sharp natural Cheddar cheese,
  shredded

1. Pour buttermilk over bran in small bowl; let stand until softened.
2. Cream shortening and sugar until light and fluffy.
3. Beat in egg.
4. Sift flour, baking powder, salt, and soda.
5. Add shredded cheese.
6. Fill greased muffin pans ⅔ full.
7. Bake at 400°F for about 30 minutes.
8. Serve warm.

Yield: 12 servings; *serving:* 1 muffin.

Carbohydrate, 14.9 grams; Protein, 4.3 grams; Fat, 4.8 grams.
Calories, 120 per serving.

Lemon Bread

1 cup granulated sugar
6 tablespoons vegetable
  shortening
2 eggs
½ cup milk
1½ teaspoons baking powder

Grated rind of 1 lemon
½ teaspoon salt
1½ cups flour
½ cup nuts, chopped fine

1. Cream sugar and shortening.
2. Add eggs and milk.
3. Combine flour, salt, and baking powder.
4. Add flour mixture to the creamed sugar mixture.
5. Add lemon rind and chopped nuts.
6. Mix until smooth.
7. Pour mixture into 8-inch loaf pan.
8. Bake at 300° or 325°F for 45 minutes to 1 hour.
9. While warm, pour sauce over bread. See recipe below for sauce.

Sauce for Lemon Bread

Juice of 1 lemon
¼ cup sugar

1. Mix lemon juice and sugar.
2. Cook to syrup stage (not until sticky).
3. Pour sauce over lemon bread.

Yield: 1 loaf (14 slices).

Carbohydrate, 24.3 grams; Protein, 3.0 grams; Fat, 9.5 grams.
Calories, 195 per slice.

Fiesta-Banana Bread

1 cup bananas, mashed
2 cups flour, sifted
1 teaspoon baking powder
1 teaspoon soda
¾ teaspoon salt
½ cup vegetable shortening
1½ cups sugar
2 eggs, unbeaten
1 teaspoon vanilla
½ cup buttermilk or sour milk
1 cup walnuts, finely ground

1. Combine shortening, sugar, eggs, and vanilla, and beat for 2 minutes.
2. Add buttermilk and flour mixture alternately with mashed bananas.
3. Beat long enough to blend.
4. Add ground walnuts.
5. Bake at 350°F for 1 hour.

Yield: 1 loaf (14 slices).

Carbohydrate, 38.2 grams; Protein, 4.2 grams; Fat, 7.7 grams.
Calories, 239 per slice.

Whole-Wheat Pancakes

1 egg
1 cup buttermilk
2 tablespoons melted
  shortening or oil
¾ cup whole-wheat flour
1 tablespoon granulated or brown
  sugar
1 teaspoon baking powder
½ teaspoon soda
½ teaspoon salt

1. Beat egg; add remaining ingredients in order listed, and beat with rotary beater until smooth.
2. Spray heated griddle with Pam.
3. Pour ¼ cup of batter on iron for each pancake.
4. Turn pancakes as soon as they are puffed and edges begin to dry slightly.
5. Bake other side until golden brown.

Yield: 10 servings; *serving:* 1 pancake.

Carbohydrate, 17.3 grams; Protein, 5.4 grams; Fat, 7.8 grams.
Calories, 161 per serving.

Soybean Waffles

2¼ cups water
1½ cups rolled oats
1 tablespoon oil

1 cup soaked soybeans
½ teaspoon salt

1. Soak soybeans several hours or overnight; keep covered with water.
2. Drain; discard water.
3. Combine all ingredients and blend until light and foamy—about half a minute.
4. Let stand while waffle iron is heating.
5. After the waffle batter thickens on standing, blend it briefly and pour into a pitcher for convenience.
6. Spray iron with Pam to prevent sticking.
7. Pour batter in hot waffle iron and bake for 11–12 minutes.
8. Do not open iron before time is up.

Yield: 10 servings.

Carbohydrate, 31.2 grams; Protein, 17.4 grams; Fat, 12.1 grams.
Calories, 304 per serving.

Wheat Sticks

1 cup whole-wheat flour
¾ cup unbleached flour
2 tablespoons soy flour
¼ cup wheat germ

1 teaspoon salt
6 tablespoons oil
6 tablespoons water
1 tablespoon brown sugar

1. Mix dry ingredients.
2. Add oil and mix as for pie crust.
3. Add water and knead thoroughly.
4. Roll thin and put on cookie sheet.
5. Cut in strips and bake at 325°F until lightly browned.

Yield: 5 dozen; *serving:* 3 sticks.

Carbohydrate, 8.9 grams; Protein, 1.9 grams; Fat, 4.7 grams.
Calories, 86 per serving.

Whole-Wheat Crackers

4 cups whole-wheat pastry
   flour
⅔ cup margarine
2 teaspoons salt

1 cup sugar
1¼ cup walnuts, finely ground
1 cup water
1 tablespoon oil

1. Mix all ingredients together.
2. Divide dough in half. Roll out each half on large, oiled cookie sheet.
3. Take a knife and mark out each cracker.
4. Bake at 325°F for 15 minutes.

Yield: 100 crackers.

Carbohydrate, 5.4 grams; Protein, .5 gram; Fat, 2 grams.
Calories, 42 per cracker.

Yeast Corn Bread

2 tablespoons dry yeast
1 cup warm water
½ teaspoon honey
5 cups warm water
2½ cups corn meal
2 tablespoons honey

3 teaspoons salt
½ cup potato flakes
2 tablespoons oil
3 eggs
2 tablespoons powdered milk or
   buttermilk
9–10 cups unbleached flour

1. Combine dry yeast, 1 cup warm water, and ½ teaspoon honey.
2. Mix and let stand to dissolve the yeast.
3. Combine the next eight ingredients and mix thoroughly.
4. Add the dissolved yeast mixture and mix well.
5. Add the unbleached flour (a cup at a time), and knead well. Work until the dough is smooth and elastic.
6. Place in an oiled bowl. Cover and let rise until double in size (1 to 1½ hours).
7. Punch down and knead about one minute.
8. Shape into loaves.
9. Place in lightly oiled 8-inch pans.
10. Cover and let rise until the dough swells just over the top of the pan.
11. Bake in preheated oven for 10 minutes at 425°F and then reduce the heat to 350°F and bake for 25 minutes. (May be baked in clay flower pots.)

Yield: 4 loaves (15 slices/loaf); *serving:* 1 slice.

Carbohydrate, 19.5 grams; Protein, 3.1 grams; Fat, 1 gram.
Calories, 102 per serving.

Pecan Rolls

1 package dry yeast
¼ cup warm water
½ cup milk
¼ cup sugar
½ teaspoon salt
2 tablespoons shortening, melted

2½ cups unbleached flour, sifted
1 egg
2 tablespoons honey
¼ cup brown sugar
½ cup pecan pieces
1 teaspoon oil
2 tablespoons margarine

1. Dissolve yeast in warm water.
2. Scald milk; pour milk into large mixing bowl of electric mixer.
3. Add sugar, salt, and shortening. Cool until just warm.
4. Stir in one half of the flour. Mix in dissolved yeast.
5. Add egg and beat well.
6. Stir in remaining flour and knead, adding more flour if needed to make soft dough.
7. Knead until dough is smooth and satiny (approximately 5 minutes).
8. Shape into smooth ball.
9. Wash mixing bowl, then oil lightly. Roll dough in bowl to oil dough lightly.
10. Punch dough down. Cover and let rise 5 to 10 minutes.
11. Roll out dough to ¼-inch thickness. Spread with margarine, then sprinkle with sugar and cinnamon mixture, also nuts if desired.
12. Roll up dough as a jelly roll. Slice in ½-inch to 1-inch slices.
13. Drizzle honey over buttered pans. Sprinkle brown sugar, pecan pieces or nutmeats as desired, on top of mixture.
14. Place sliced dough on top of mixture and let rise until doubled in bulk.
15. Bake at 350°F for 25 to 30 minutes.

Yield: 1 dozen rolls.

Carbohydrate, 27.2 grams; Protein, 3.6 grams; Fat, 6.3 grams.
Calories, 189 per serving.

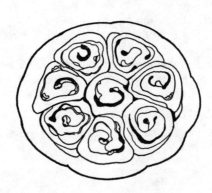

Dilly Bread

1 package yeast	1 tablespoon instant minced onion
¼ cup warm water	2 teaspoons dillseed
1 cup creamed cottage	1 egg
cheese (heated to lukewarm)	2½ cups unbleached flour
1 tablespoon margarine	
1 teaspoon salt	

1. Soften yeast in water. Let stand 10 minutes.
2. Combine in large bowl all ingredients, except flour, adding yeast last, then add flour.
3. Cover, let rise until doubled in bulk.
4. Stir down, then turn into oiled casserole.
5. Let rise again.
6. Bake at 350°F for 45 minutes.
7. May brush top with margarine and sprinkle with salt.

Yield: 1 loaf (14 slices).

Carbohydrate, 16.5 grams; Protein, 5.6 grams; Fat, 2.1 grams.
Calories, 108 per serving.

Rye Bread

2 tablespoons yeast	1½ tablespoons honey
½ cup warm water	2 tablespoons molasses
½ teaspoon honey	2 teaspoons salt
2 cups warm water	2 cups rye flour
1 cup potato flakes	3 cups unbleached flour

1. Combine dry yeast, ½ cup warm water, and ½ teaspoon honey.
2. Mix and set aside to dissolve the yeast.
3. Combine the next six ingredients, mixing thoroughly.
4. Add the dissolved yeast mixture and mix well.
5. Add the unbleached flour (a cup at a time), and knead well. Work until the dough is smooth and elastic (may be a little sticky).
6. Place in an oiled bowl, cover and let rise until double in size (1 to 1½ hours).
7. Punch down and knead about one minute.
8. Shape into loaves.
9. Place in lightly oiled 8-inch pans.
10. Cover and let rise until the dough swells just over the top of pan.
11. Bake in preheated oven for 10 minutes at 425°F. Then reduce heat to 350°F and continue baking for 25 minutes.

Yield: 2 loaves (15 slices/loaf); *serving:* 1 slice.

Carbohydrate, 15.7 grams; Protein, 2.2 grams; Fat, .4 gram.
Calories, 75 per serving.

Potato Bread

2 tablespoons dry yeast	¼ cup oil
½ cup warm water	2 teaspoons salt
½ teaspoon honey	¾ cup whole-wheat flour
2½ cups warm water	8–9 cups unbleached flour
1 cup potato flakes	

1. Combine dry yeast, ½ cup warm water, and ½ teaspoon honey. Mix and let stand to dissolve the yeast.
2. Combine the next five ingredients and mix thoroughly.
3. Add the dissolved yeast mixture and mix well.
4. Add the unbleached flour (a cup at a time), and knead well. Work until the dough is smooth and elastic.
5. Place in an oiled bowl. Cover and let rise until double in size (1 to 1½ hours).
6. Punch down and knead about one minute.
7. Shape into loaves.
8. Place in lightly oiled 8-inch pans.
9. Cover and let rise until the dough swells just over top of pan.
10. Bake in preheated oven for 10 minutes at 425°F and then reduce the heat to 350°F and bake for 25 minutes.

Yield: 4 loaves (15 slices/loaf); *serving:* 1 slice.

Carbohydrate, 15 grams; Protein, 2.5 grams; Fat, 1.2 grams. Calories, 82 per serving.

Seven-Grain Bread

1–1½ tablespoons dry yeast	1 tablespoon honey
½ cup warm water	2 tablespoons molasses
½ teaspoon honey	2 teaspoons salt
2 cups warm water	1½ cups seven-grain cereal
2 cups unbleached flour	3–4 cups unbleached flour (could
2 tablespoons oil	substitute 1 cup whole-wheat flour)

1. Combine dry yeast, ½ cup warm water, and ½ teaspoon honey.
2. Mix and let stand to dissolve the yeast.
3. Combine the next seven ingredients and mix thoroughly.
4. Add the dissolved yeast mixture and mix well.
5. Add the unbleached flour (a cup at a time), and knead well. Work until the dough is smooth and elastic.
6. Place in an oiled bowl. Cover and let rise until double in size (1 to 1½ hours).
7. Punch down and knead about one minute.
8. Shape into loaves.
9. Place in lightly oiled 8-inch pans.
10. Cover and let rise until the dough swells just over top of pan.
11. Bake in preheated oven for 10 minutes at 425°F and then reduce the heat to 350°F and bake for 25 minutes.

Yield: 2 loaves (15 slices/loaf); *serving:* 1 slice.

Carbohydrate, 10.6 grams; Protein, 1.7 grams; Fat, .4 gram. Calories, 53 per serving.

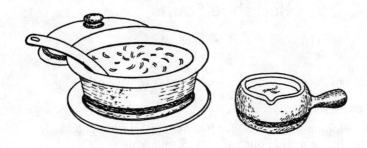

Wholesome Soups

Soups served hot at the beginning of the meal stimulate the digestive juices. Soups are easily made, economical, and, when properly prepared, are a very desirable food in the diet.

Soups may also be used as the main course. Some soups can incorporate vegetables and protein to make them a full meal. Chowders and stews are examples.

Soups may be colorful and served in a very attractive manner. They may be enhanced by adding a favorite garnish—seeds, nuts, bread crumbs, croutons, chopped parsley, watercress, grated cheese, herbs, or sliced, hard-boiled eggs.

Save vegetable cooking water to be added to soup, thus providing additional nutrients and enhancing flavor.

Bean Soup

½ cup plus 2 tablespoons
 navy beans
1½ teaspoons oil
3 cups cold water
½ teaspoon salt
1 tablespoon beef-like
 seasoning (see p. 174)

4 teaspoons onions, dehydrated
⅓ cup carrots, diced
½ cup potatoes, diced
¼ cup celery, chopped fine

1. Sort and wash beans, place with oil and water in pan, and cook until about ¾ done (approximately 1 hour).
2. Add salt, beef-like seasoning, onions, carrots, potatoes, and celery.
3. Continue cooking until done (approximately 30 minutes).
4. Mix well and place in dish to serve.

Note: To puree, place in blender.

Yield: 10 servings.

Carbohydrate, 10.6 grams; Protein, 3.2 grams; Fat, 0.9 gram.
Calories, 63 per serving.

Berkshire Soup

1 onion, chopped fine
¼ cup margarine
½ bay leaf
2 tablespoons flour
4 cups canned tomatoes
2 tablespoons sugar

1 teaspoon salt
2 cups boiling water
2 cups canned corn
½ cup cream or half-and-half
2 egg yolks

1. Cook onion and margarine for five minutes, stirring constantly.
2. Add the bay leaf and flour and cook 2 minutes.
3. Add tomatoes, sugar, salt, and boiling water.
4. Simmer 20 minutes.
5. Add corn and cook 10 minutes.
6. Press through a strainer.
7. Just before serving, add yolks of eggs, slightly beaten and diluted with cream.

Yield: 12 servings.

Carbohydrate, 20.5 grams; Protein, 3.4 grams; Fat, 6.5 grams.
Calories, 154 per serving.

Boston Potato Chowder

¾ cup potatoes, diced
2 teaspoons onions,
  dehydrated
3 tablespoons celery,
  chopped fine
1⅓ cups water
3 tablespoons mushroom
  pieces, canned

2½ cups Medium White Sauce (see
  p. 175)
¾ teaspoon chicken-like seasoning
  (see p. 174)
½ teaspoon salt
1 tablespoon cornstarch
2 tablespoons water

1. Place potatoes, onions, celery, and water in pan, and cook until tender.
2. Chop mushrooms fine.
3. Combine vegetables, mushrooms, and white sauce.
4. Combine cornstarch and water, add to cooked vegetables.
5. Add chicken-like seasoning and salt. Heat.
6. Serve hot.

Yield: 10 servings.

Carbohydrate, 13.5 grams; Protein, 3.0 grams; Fat, 2.8 grams.
Calories, 91 per serving.

Boundary Castle Soup

1 cup tomatoes
¾ cup chopped mushrooms
¼ cup chopped onions
1 tablespoon chopped parsley
1 tablespoon flour

1 tablespoon margarine
1 cup milk
½ cup cream or half-and-half
1 teaspoon salt

1. Brown the mushrooms and onions in the margarine.
2. Add the flour and tomatoes, and bring to a boil.
3. Add the cream and milk.
4. Reheat. Add salt and parsley.

Yield: 6 servings.

Carbohydrate, 6.5 grams; Protein, 2.8 grams; Fat, 5.8 grams.
Calories, 89 per serving.

Chicken-like Broth—Vegetarian

2 onions, finely chopped
4 stalks celery
1 green pepper
2 tablespoons margarine
¼ cup parsley, chopped
1 cup nutmeats, chopped

4 tablespoons flour
1 can asparagus
3 quarts water
1 tablespoon Vegex (see p. 174)
Salt to taste

1. Cook onions, celery, and green pepper in margarine until brown.
2. Add parsley, nutmeats, and flour. Cook 5 minutes.
3. Add asparagus and water. Boil 15 minutes.
4. Strain through colander.
5. Season with Vegex and salt.
6. Reheat and serve.

Yield: 8 1-cup servings.

Carbohydrate, 10.5 grams; Protein, 5.7 grams; Fat, 7.6 grams.
Calories, 134 per serving.

Chili Bean Soup

¾ cup pinto beans
2 cups water
¾ cup diced tomatoes, canned
½ cup plus 2 tablespoons tomato sauce, canned
½ teaspoon onions dehydrated
½ teaspoon green peppers, dehydrated
Salt to taste
1 teaspoon chili powder
Dash garlic powder
Dash cornstarch

1. Sort beans, making sure they are clean of particles, and wash thoroughly.
2. Cook beans in water until tender.
3. Add the rest of the ingredients except cornstarch.
4. Simmer for 1 hour.
5. Thicken with cornstarch when done.

Yield: 10 servings.

Carbohydrate, 30.4 grams; Protein, 10.0 grams; Fat, 1.8 grams.
Calories, 181 per serving

Colonial Soup

¼ cup carrot, grated
½ cup potatoes
1 small onion, finely diced
2 tablespoons margarine
3 cups water
½ bay leaf
½ cup bread cubes, very small
1 egg
1 tablespoon water
Salt to taste

1. Pare and grate carrots, potatoes, and onion.
2. Put 2 tablespoons margarine in soup kettle.
3. Add vegetables, then brown.
4. Add water, bay leaf, and salt.
5. Let simmer for 30 minutes.
6. Beat the egg well. Add tablespoon water.
7. Pour mixture over the bread, making sure each cube is well-coated.
8. Drop into the soup kettle.
9. Bring to a boil and serve.

Yield: 6 servings.

Carbohydrate, 11.6 grams; Protein, 2.7 grams; Fat, 5.0 grams.
Calories, 102 per serving.

Corn Chowder with Imitation Baco-Bits

⅓ cup whole-kernel corn
⅓ cup potatoes, diced
¼ cup celery, chopped
¾ cup cream-style corn, canned
½ cup plus 5 teaspoons non-fat milk

3 cups Thin White Sauce (see p. 175)
Dash onion powder
¼ teaspoon parsley, dehydrated
½ teaspoon imitation baco-bits (see p. 174)
1 teaspoon salt

1. Place potatoes and celery in kettle with small amount of water and cook until done.
2. Combine potatoes, celery, cream-style corn, and milk in kettle.
3. Add onion powder, imitation baco-bits, and parsley to mixture. Stir well and heat.
4. Add white sauce, salt.
5. Stir well and heat.

Yield: 10 servings.

Carbohydrate, 11.8 grams; Protein, 4.0 grams; Fat, .2 gram.
Calories, 65 per serving.

English Barley Soup

1 cup water
2½ tablespoons barley
1 tablespoon oil
3¼ cups water
½ cup split peas

¼ teaspoon oil
3 tablespoons onion, chopped
½ teaspoon salt
2 teaspoons chicken-like seasoning (see p. 174)

1. Rinse barley and soak overnight in 1 cup water.
2. Cook barley in soaking water and 1 tablespoon oil until tender.
3. Cook split peas, onion, 3¼ cups water, and ¼ teaspoon oil until tender.
4. Puree peas if necessary.
5. Combine peas, barley, salt, and chicken-like seasoning.
6. Heat and serve.

Yield: 10 servings.

Carbohydrate, 6.6 grams; Protein, 1.7 grams; Fat, .3 gram.
Calories, 35 per serving.

French Onion Soup

1 tablespoon margarine
1¼ cups onions, diced
3 cups water
1 teaspoon beef-flavor
seasoning (see p. 174)

1 teaspoon chicken-like seasoning
(see p. 174)
½ teaspoon salt

1. Sauté onions in margarine in uncovered pan until onions begin to brown an even color.
2. Add water and seasonings.
3. Bring to boil and simmer for about 25 minutes or until onion flavor is well developed.

Yield: 10 servings.

Carbohydrate, 1.6 grams; Protein, .3 gram; Fat, 1.1 grams.
Calories, 17 per serving

Golden Bouillon

1 large onion
1 turnip
1 potato
1 cup shredded cabbage
4 carrots

4 stalks celery
1 bell pepper
Salt to taste
1 tablespoon margarine
2 tablespoons Savorex (see p. 174)

1. Cook vegetables in 1 gallon of water until tender.
2. Strain through colander.
3. Add salt, 1 tablespoon of margarine, and 2 tablespoons of Savorex.
4. Reheat and serve.

Yield: 8 servings.

Carbohydrate, 11.5 grams; Protein, 1.7 grams; Fat, 1.7 grams.
Calories, 68 per serving.

Hungarian Vegetable Stew

¼ cup vegetable oil
3 large onions, chopped
4 green peppers, seeded and
cut into strips

3 tomatoes, washed and diced
1 eggplant, peeled and diced
Salt to taste

1. Heat oil in heavy skillet and sauté the onions until tender.
2. Add green peppers, tomatoes, and eggplant.
3. Bring to a boil, season with salt, cover and simmer until vegetables are tender (about 20 minutes).

Yield: 6 servings of 1 cup each.

Carbohydrate, 15.1 grams; Protein, 2.9 grams; Fat, 3.9 grams.
Calories, 108 per serving.

Lentil Pottage

⅓ cup rice
4 cups water
1 teaspoon salt
1 cup sautéed onions

2 tablespoons oil
1 cup lentils
parsley, red pepper, or pimento for garnish

1. Add rice to boiling salted water.
2. Cover. Cook 15 minutes.
3. Add onions, oil, and lentils.
4. Boil until lentils are tender—consistency of mush.
5. Garnish with parsley and slices of red pepper or pimento.
6. Serve hot.

Yield: 6 servings of ½ cup each.

Carbohydrate, 17.2 grams; Protein, 3.6 grams; Fat, 5.2 grams. Calories, 130 per serving.

Lentil and Rice Soup

½ cup lentils
2 cups water
⅓ cup natural rice
1 small onion

1 teaspoon salt
1½ tablespoons margarine
1 tablespoon flour
½ cup evaporated milk

1. Cook lentils in two cups of water until partially done.
2. Add rice, onion, salt, and cook until tender.
3. Melt margarine and blend with flour.
4. Stir into lentils and rice.
5. Add milk, mixing well.
6. Heat and serve.

Yield: 6 servings of ½ cup each.

Carbohydrate, 9.4 grams; Protein, 3.3 grams; Fat, 5.5 grams. Calories, 100 per serving.

Potato Chowder

¾ cup potatoes, diced
¼ cup celery, diced
1½ cups water
2½ cups Thin White Sauce (see p. 175)

1 teaspoon chicken-like seasoning (see p. 174)
½ teaspoon salt

1. Place potatoes, celery, and water in kettle, and cook until done.
2. Combine vegetables with white sauce in kettle.
3. Add seasonings to white sauce mixture and heat.
4. To puree, use blender.

Yield: 10 servings.

Carbohydrate, 13.1 grams; Protein, 3.1 grams; Fat, 2.8 grams. Calories, 90 per serving.

Pottage Germain

2 cups potatoes, diced	2 tablespoons margarine
3 stalks celery	2 cups green peas
6 cups cold water	1 small onion, diced
1 cup whole milk	1 teaspoon salt

1. Cook celery, potatoes, onion, and margarine in water until tender.
2. Add peas, then put through colander.
3. Add 1 cup whole milk, and salt.
4. Reheat and serve.

Yield: 10 servings.

Carbohydrate, 9.4 grams; Protein, 2.3 grams; Fat, 3.2 grams. Calories, 76 per serving.

Scotch Barley Soup

1 cup pearl barley	1 stalk diced celery
6 carrots, grated	2 cups chopped cabbage
4 potatoes, diced	2 cups tomatoes
2 large onions	Salt to taste
6 quarts water	1 teaspoon Savorex (see p. 174)

1. Cook vegetables in water 45 minutes.
2. Add barley and cook 30 minutes longer.
3. Add margarine, Savorex, and salt.

Yield: 10 servings.

Carbohydrate, 33.7 grams; Protein, 4.3 grams; Fat, 9.6 grams. Calories, 239 per serving.

Split Pea Soup

¾ cup split peas	¼ cup carrots, diced
1½ teaspoons onions, dehydrated	½ teaspoon beef-like seasoning (see p. 174)
3½ cups water	1 teaspoon torumel yeast
1 cup potatoes	½ teaspoon salt
½ cup celery, chopped fine	

1. Wash split peas.
2. Place peas and onions with water in a pan. Bring to boiling, and cook for 45 minutes.
3. Add all remaining ingredients, and cook 20 minutes more.
4. Place in blender and puree.
5. Heat and serve.

Yield: 10 servings.

Carbohydrate, 12.8 grams; Protein, 4.0 grams; Fat, .2 gram. Calories, 67 per serving.

Tomato Broth with Barley

4 cups canned or fresh
  tomatoes
2 tablespoons sliced onion
2 stalks celery, cut up
1 bay leaf
Sprig of parsley, chopped fine

1 quart of water
¼ cup pearl barley
2 cups water
1 tablespoon margarine
Salt to taste

1. Mix tomatoes, onion, celery, bay leaf, and parsley.
2. Add 1 quart of water, let boil 45 minutes, then strain.
3. Cook pearl barley in 2 cups water and margarine until done.
4. Add the barley to the tomato broth.
5. Salt to taste, and serve hot.

Yield: 4 servings.

Carbohydrate, 21.1 grams; Protein, 3.5 grams; Fat, 3.4 grams.
Calories, 129 per serving.

Vegetable Soup

1 cup mixed vegetables,
  frozen
¼ cup potatoes, diced
¼ cup carrots, diced
¼ cup celery, diced
3½ cups water
½ cup tomatoes, diced,
  canned

½ cup cream of tomato soup
½ teaspoon salt
½ teaspoon yeast extract
½ teaspoon chicken-like seasoning
  (see p. 174)
½ teaspoon sugar

1. Heat water; add all vegetables and seasonings.
2. Bring to a boil.
3. Simmer 1½ to 2 hours.
4. Serve hot.

Note: To puree, place in blender; strain.

Yield: 10 servings.

Carbohydrate, 3.3 grams; Protein, .8 gram; Fat, .2 gram.
Calories, 18 per serving.

Washington Chowder

¾ cup potatoes, diced
¼ cup celery, diced
2¾ cups low-fat milk
½ cup tomatoes, diced,
  canned
1 cup corn

1 teaspoon salt
Dash chicken-like seasoning (see
  p. 174)
1 teaspoon cornstarch
1 tablespoon water

1. Cook potatoes and celery until tender.
2. Add cooked vegetables, tomatoes, corn, cornstarch, and seasonings.
3. Heat and serve hot.

Yield: 10 servings.

Carbohydrate, 9.3 grams; Protein, 3.7 grams; Fat, .8 gram.
Calories, 58 per serving.

Asparagus Cream Soup

7¾ ounces asparagus spears, frozen   4¼ cups Thin White Sauce (see p. 175)
½ teaspoon salt

1. Cook asparagus in small amount of water until tender.
2. Place asparagus in blender and puree.
3. Combine asparagus, white sauce, and salt. Mix well.
4. Heat together before serving.

Yield: 10 servings.

Carbohydrate, 12.3 grams; Protein, 7.9 grams; Fat, 4.8 grams.
Calories, 121 per serving.

Avocado Cream Soup

¼ cup pearl barley
1 quart water
½ cup chopped celery or celery leaves
1 small onion
Few sprigs of parsley

1 bay leaf
1 medium avocado, put through fine sieve
2 egg yolks (beaten)
1 cup thin cream
Salt to taste

1. Cook pearl barley in water for 1 hour.
2. Add celery, onion, parsley, salt, bay leaf.
3. Cook ½ hour longer.
4. Mix avocado and egg yolks, and combine with broth.
5. Place mixture in double boiler for a few minutes and stir.
6. Just before serving add the cream.

Yield: 10 servings.

Carbohydrate, 7.1 grams; Protein, 2.3 grams; Fat, 9.7 grams.
Calories, 121 per serving.

Barley Cream Soup

¼ cup barley
1½ cups water
¼ cup potatoes
¼ cup celery, chopped

2½ cups Thin White Sauce (see p. 175)
2 teaspoons onion powder

1. Cook barley with water for 1 hour.
2. Cook potatoes and celery until tender.
3. Combine barley, potatoes, and celery with white sauce.
4. Add onion powder to white sauce mixture. Stir well.
5. Heat before serving.

Yield: 10 servings.

Carbohydrate, 6.6 grams; Protein, 1.7 grams; Fat, .3 gram.
Calories, 35 per serving.

Broccoli Cream Soup

½ cup potatoes
½ cup celery, chopped
1½ tablespoons onions, chopped
3½ cups low-fat milk

¾ cup broccoli spears, puree
1 teaspoon salt
1 teaspoon chicken-like seasoning (see p. 174)

1. Cook the potatoes, celery, and onions in small amount of water for 25 minutes.
2. Puree and strain.
3. Cook broccoli in small amount of water until tender, puree and strain.
4. Heat milk, add pureed vegetables, salt, and chicken-like seasoning.
5. Heat and serve. *Do not boil.*

Yield: 10 servings.

Carbohydrate, 7.3 grams; Protein, 4.2 grams; Fat, .9 gram.
Calories, 51 per serving.

Carrot Cream Soup

2 cups grated carrots
3 cups milk
1 medium onion, sliced
2 tablespoons margarine

2 tablespoons flour
1 tablespoon salt
Cold water as needed

1. Add carrots to the milk and heat in double boiler.
2. Add sliced onion and cook 10 minutes.
3. Remove onion. Mix flour and salt in a little water, and stir into hot milk.
4. Add margarine.

Yield: 6 servings.

Carbohydrate, 14.0 grams; Protein, 6.0 grams; Fat, 6.4 grams.
Calories, 136 per serving.

Chicken Cream Soup—Vegetarian

1 cup chopped onion
½ cup celery
½ cup parsley
½ cup green pepper
2 tablespoons margarine
4 cups milk
½ cup cream

¼ cup nut meats, diced
1 egg
3 tablespoons flour
2 tablespoons milk
Salt to taste
1 tablespoon Vegex (see p. 174)

1. Cook onion, celery, parsley, green pepper in margarine until golden brown.
2. Add 2 tablespoons of flour and brown slightly.
3. Add 4 cups of milk and ½ cup cream. Bring to boil.
4. Add ¼ cup diced nut meats.
5. Mix egg, 1 tablespoon of flour, and 2 tablespoons of milk.
6. Drop batter into hot soup. Do not stir for a few minutes.
7. Let cook for 5 minutes.
8. Add salt and Vegex. Serve at once.

Yield: 12 servings.

Carbohydrate, 8.3 grams; Protein, 5.2 grams; Fat, 6.9 grams.
Calories, 125 per serving.

Cheese Cream Soup

2½ tablespoons margarine
1 teaspoon onion powder
1 tablespoon plus 1 teaspoon
  flour
2¼ cups low-fat milk
1¾ cups water
Dash paprika
½ teaspoon salt

Dash chili powder
2 teaspoons chicken-like seasoning
  (see p. 174)
1 tablespoon plus ½ teaspoon parsley,
  dehydrated
¼ cup carrots, diced
3 slices American cheese
Dash celery salt

1. Melt margarine and blend in onion powder.
2. Blend in flour, and cook for 3 to 4 minutes.
3. Place milk and water in pan, and heat for 10 minutes.
4. Add heated milk/water mixture to flour mixture. Cook until thickened while stirring constantly.
5. Add paprika, salt, chili powder, chicken-like seasoning, celery salt, and parsley. Mix well.
6. Cook carrots in small amount of water until tender.
7. Add carrots to mixture and mix well.
8. Add cheese just before serving. Stir until blended.

Yield: 10 servings.

Carbohydrate, 6.1 grams; Protein, 4.3 grams; Fat, 5.5 grams.
Calories, 91 per serving.

Corn Cream Soup

1½ cups cream-style corn, canned   3¼ cups Thin White Sauce (see p. 175)

1. Place corn in blender. Puree and strain.
2. Place corn and white sauce in pan, and heat.

Yield: 10 servings.

Carbohydrate, 13.4 grams; Protein, 3.9 grams; Fat, .2 gram.
Calories, 69 per serving.

Green-Bean Cream Soup

3½ cups low-fat milk
2½ tablespoons margarine
1 tablespoon flour

1 teaspoon salt
1¼ cup green beans, cut, frozen

1. Heat milk.
2. Melt margarine, then add flour and salt.
3. Mix margarine and flour mixture with hot milk, stirring briskly until smooth and thickened.
4. Cook green beans in small amount of water until tender. Puree.
5. Blend with white sauce.
6. Heat and serve.

Yield: 10 servings.

Carbohydrate, 7.6 grams; Protein, 4.2 grams; Fat, 3.5 grams.
Calories, 78 per serving.

Lettuce Cream Soup

4 cups milk, hot
2 tablespoons margarine, melted
4 teaspoons flour

½ teaspoon chicken-like seasoning (see p. 174)
1 teaspoon salt
¾ cup Boston lettuce, finely chopped

1. Make a thin white sauce with the first three ingredients. Add seasonings.
2. Add the chopped lettuce.
3. Heat and serve.

Yield: 10 servings.

Carbohydrate, 6.7 grams; Protein, 4.1 grams; Fat, 5.8 grams.
Calories, 96 per serving.

Leek Cream Soup

2 tablespoons oil
1 bunch leeks
1 quart broth (water + 1 tablespoon chicken-like seasoning [see p. 174])

2 medium potatoes
2 tablespoons parsley, minced
1 can condensed milk
Salt to taste

1. Wash leeks carefully, slitting down sides to be sure all grit is washed out.
2. Slice leeks.
3. Braise leeks slowly in the oil for 5 minutes.
4. Peel and slice potatoes.
5. Add broth and potatoes. Simmer 20 minutes or until potatoes are tender.
6. Add salt to taste, parsley, and canned milk.
7. Reheat. Serve as is or put through blender.

Yield: 8 servings of ½ cup each.

Carbohydrate, 26.4 grams; Protein, 4.0 grams; Fat, 7.0 grams.
Calories, 185 per serving.

Lentil Cream Soup

1½ cups lentils, cooked
⅔ cup water
2¼ cups low-fat milk
½ teaspoon salt

½ cup celery, diced
¾ cup potatoes, diced
1 teaspoon chicken-flavor seasoning (see p. 174)

1. Puree and strain cooked lentils.
2. Cook celery and potatoes in small amount of water.
3. Heat milk with cooked celery and potatoes.
4. Add salt, chicken-flavor seasoning, and lentils.
5. Cook until tender. Serve hot.

Yield: 10 servings.

Carbohydrate, 10.7 grams; Protein, 4.7 grams; Fat, .6 gram.
Calories, 66 per serving

Navy Bean Cream Soup

½ cup water
⅓ cup navy beans
¼ teaspoon oil
1 tablespoon cornstarch

2¾ cups low-fat milk
1 cup cream or half-and-half
1 teaspoon salt

1. Sort and wash beans. Soak overnight in ½ cup water.
2. Add oil to the soaked beans and water.
3. Cook until tender.
4. Puree and strain.
5. Mix cornstarch with a small amount of milk.
6. Heat remaining milk and half-and-half.
7. Add cornstarch mixture, stirring until cornstarch is cooked.
8. Add bean puree, salt.
9. Heat and serve.

Yield: 10 servings.

Carbohydrate, 17.7 grams; Protein, 4.1 grams; Fat, 1.0 gram.
Calories, 92 per serving.

Olive Cream Soup

¾ cup celery, finely chopped
1 cup potatoes
3½ tablespoons black olives,
  finely chopped

2¾ cups low-fat milk
1½ teaspoons salt
1 teaspoon chicken-like seasoning
  (see p. 174)

1. Cook celery and potatoes in small amount of water until tender.
2. Puree and strain.
3. Add olives, milk, salt, chicken-like seasoning.
4. Heat and serve.

Yield: 10 servings.

Carbohydrate, 8.1 grams; Protein, 3.5 grams; Fat, .7 gram.
Calories, 53 per serving.

Pea Cream Soup

1¼ cups green peas frozen
3 cups Thin White Sauce (see p. 175)
½ teaspoon salt
½ teaspoon chicken-like seasoning (see p. 174)
1 tablespoon plus 1 teaspoon flour

1. Cook peas in very small amount of water.
2. Place peas in blender and puree, then strain.
3. Combine peas, white sauce, seasoning, and flour in a pan. Mix well.
4. Heat and serve.

Yield: 10 servings.

Carbohydrate, 12.0 grams; Protein, 5.2 grams; Fat, .1 gram. Calories, 71 per serving.

Potato Cream Soup

2 cups potatoes, diced
½ cup celery, diced
½ teaspoon salt
½ teaspoon chicken-like seasoning (see p. 174)
3½ cups low-fat milk

1. Cook potatoes and celery in small amount of water until tender.
2. Add milk and heat.
3. Add salt. Stir to blend.
4. Strain.
5. Heat before serving.

Yield: 10 servings.

Carbohydrate, 8.4 grams; Protein, 4.1 grams; Fat, .9 gram. Calories, 58 per serving.

Spinach Cream Soup

3¼ cups low-fat milk
2 tablespoons margarine, melted
1 tablespoon flour
1 teaspoon salt
1¼ cups spinach, frozen

1. Cook spinach in small amount of water, and puree.
2. Heat milk.
3. Melt margarine and mix with flour.
4. Add to hot milk, stirring briskly.
5. Add salt.
6. Cook until smooth and of thin consistency.
7. Add spinach puree.
8. Heat and serve.

Yield: 10 servings.

Carbohydrate, 6.4 grams; Protein, 3.9 grams; Fat, 3.4 grams. Calories, 70 per serving.

Vegetable Cream Soup

2 cups mixed vegetables,
  frozen
½ cup celery, diced
1 tablespoon onions,
  dehydrated
½ cup potatoes, diced
3½ tablespoons V-8 juice,
  canned

1 teaspoon salt
½ teaspoon beef-like seasoning (see
  p. 174)
1 cup water
2 cups low-fat milk

1. Place vegetables, celery, onions, and potatoes in a pan, and cook in small amount of water until tender.
2. Puree ½ the vegetables, then combine all vegetables in a soup pot.
3. Add V-8 juice, salt, beef-like seasoning, and water to soup.
4. Add milk.
5. Heat soup but do not boil.

Yield: 10 servings.

Carbohydrate, 14.0 grams; Protein, 3.6 grams; Fat, .6 gram.
Calories, 73 per serving.

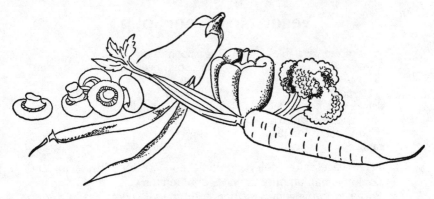

Vegetables

No foods are more universally served as part of the daily bill of fare for rich and poor alike than vegetables, and none is more frequently spoiled by overcooking.

Vegetables offer great variety in color, texture, form, and manner of preparation. They are chiefly useful because of the carbohydrates they furnish, together with an abundance of minerals, vitamins, and cellulose.

Apricot-Sweet Potato Bake

3 pounds sweet potatoes,
  baked
½ cup brown sugar
1½ tablespoons cornstarch
¼ teaspoon salt
¼ teaspoon cinnamon

2 cups canned apricots, halves
2 tablespoons grated orange peel
2 tablespoons margarine
½ cup pecans

1. Drain apricot halves and save liquid. Add water to apricot liquid to make 1 cup.
2. Mix apricot liquid, cornstarch, salt, cinnamon, and grated orange peel. Cook until thick. Cool.
3. Arrange in casserole as follows: a layer of sweet potatoes, cut lengthwise in slices ½ inch thick; a layer of apricot halves and pecan halves; sprinkle with brown sugar. Continue procedure until materials are used.
4. Cover with cooked sauce.
5. Dab the margarine on top.
6. Bake at moderate temperature until hot.

Yield: 12 servings; *serving:* ½ cup.

Carbohydrate, 41.0 grams; Protein, .2 gram; Fat, 5.0 grams.
Calories, 210 per serving.

Artichokes Supreme

12 large artichoke hearts   ½ cup mashed potatoes
½ cup peas, cooked

1. Puree peas and mix with mashed potatoes until the mixture has a consistency that can be piped through a pastry bag.
2. Season to taste and pipe through pastry bag into the artichoke hearts which have been placed on a baking pan.
3. Heat in 350°F oven for 10 minutes and serve hot.
4. Garnish with paprika or pimento slice.

Yield: 6 servings; *serving:* 2 each.

Carbohydrate, 25.0 grams; Protein, 6.8 grams; Fat, .4 gram.
Calories, 130 per serving.

Celery Amandine

2 cups celery, sliced   2 tablespoons oil or margarine
3 tablespoons almonds,   Salt to taste
   sliced

1. Sauté celery in oil or margarine until just softened.
2. Stir in almonds.
3. Salt to taste.

Yield: 6 servings; *serving:* ½ cup.

Carbohydrate, 1.7 grams; Protein, 9.0 grams; Fat, 6.4 grams.
Calories, 100 per serving.

Scalloped Corn

1 cup whole kernel corn   2 tablespoons flour
¾ cup half-and-half cream   1 teaspoon salt
¼ cup liquid from corn   3 eggs, well beaten
2 tablespoons margarine

1. Make cream sauce of margarine, flour, half-and-half cream, and corn liquid.
2. Mix corn, salt, and eggs.
3. Combine with sauce.
4. Pour into casserole and cover with bread crumbs and a dab of margarine.
5. Bake in shallow pan of water at 350°F for 45–50 minutes.

Yield: 6 servings.

Carbohydrate, 13.2 grams; Protein, 6.4 grams; Fat, 12.7 grams.
Calories, 193 per serving.

Eggplant Casserole

2 medium eggplants, fresh, diced ¾ inch
¼ cup margarine
½ cup onions, fresh, diced ½ inch
1½ cups tomatoes, diced, canned, drained (or fresh)
⅔ cup cream-of-tomato soup
½ teaspoon salt
1 cup sour cream
1 cup Cheddar cheese, shredded

1. Steam eggplant until tender and drain.
2. Sauté onions in margarine until soft.
3. Combine eggplant, onions, diced tomatoes, tomato soup, and salt.
4. Fold in sour cream; put in buttered casserole.
5. Top with shredded cheese.
6. Bake until bubbly and cheese is melted.

Yield: 10 servings.

Carbohydrate, 16.5 grams; Protein, 6.9 grams; Fat, 8.1 grams. Calories, 167 per serving.

Green Beans—Viennese Style

1½ pounds green beans
1½ tablespoons margarine
1½ tablespoons flour
½ onion, chopped
½ tablespoon dill, chopped
¼ teaspoon parsley, chopped
¼ cup bouillon
½ tablespoon lemon juice
½ cup sour cream
Dash of salt

1. Clean beans, cut off ends, and wash thoroughly.
2. Cut into small pieces and cook in small amount of salted water about 20 minutes.
3. Melt the margarine, blend in the flour, add onion and brown.
4. Add dill, parsley, and bouillon and bring to a boil.
5. Add the beans, lemon juice, dash of salt, and sour cream.
6. Bring to a boil again and serve.

Yield: 5 servings; *serving:* ½ cup.

Carbohydrate, 14.1 grams; Protein, 3.6 grams; Fat 8.9 grams. Calories, 150 per serving.

Peas and Water Chestnuts

2 cups peas (10 ounce package, frozen)
3 ounces sliced water chestnuts
2 tablespoons oil or margarine

1. Heat peas in oil or margarine until thawed.
2. Add sliced water chestnuts.
3. Continue cooking until just heated through, 2–3 minutes.

Yield: 6 servings; *serving:* ½ cup.

Carbohydrate, 9.3 grams; Protein, 2.9 grams; Fat, 5.1 grams. Calories, 95 per serving.

Stuffed Potatoes with Cottage Cheese

8 baking potatoes (medium)   1½ cups cottage cheese
1½ teaspoons salt   3 eggs
¼ cup margarine   ½ cup Cheddar cheese, grated

1. Bake potatoes in hot oven (425°F) until done.
2. Cut off top third of potatoes and scoop out potato pulp into a bowl.
3. Mash potatoes well.
4. Add salt, margarine, and cottage cheese, mixing well.
5. Add beaten eggs; beat until fluffy.
6. Spoon mixture into potato shells.
7. Sprinkle Cheddar cheese over top.
8. Return to oven (350°F) until lightly browned.

Yield: 8 servings; *serving:* 1 potato.

Carbohydrate, 19.9 grams; Protein, 14.6 grams; Fat, 11.9 grams. Calories, 245 per serving.

Squash-Filled Orange Cups

5 navel oranges, large   ½ teaspoon salt
2 pounds mashed winter   ¾ cup miniature marshmallows
  squash   ⅓ cup walnuts, chopped
5 tablespoons margarine,
  softened
3 tablespoons brown sugar

1. Cut oranges in half, removing fruit from each half.
2. Scallop edges of the shell with serrated knife blade to make cups.
3. Combine squash, margarine, brown sugar, salt, one half of the marshmallows, and walnuts. Mix well.
4. Pile mixture lightly into orange cups.
5. Top with remaining marshmallows.
6. Bake at 350°F for 15–20 minutes.

Yield: 10 servings; *serving:* ½ orange.

Carbohydrate, 19.9 grams; Protein, 2.2 grams; Fat, 9.8 grams. Calories, 177 per serving.

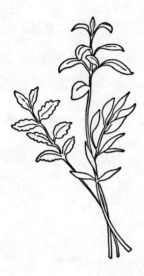

The Seasoned Art of Seasoning and Herbs Naturale

The kitchen "keyboard" is the secret of delightful cookery. Proper seasoning makes the difference. The kitchen cupboard of spices and herbs is like a "keyboard" of happy notes and harmonious flavors. A dash of this and a pinch of that suddenly makes cooking sing with flavor. Wonder-working spices and herbs give added fun and flavor to almost any food.

The use of herbs is on the increase. Herbs have a more subtle flavor than spices. An herb is the leaf of an aromatic plant which grows in the temperate zone, whereas a spice may be a root, bark, stem, leaf, bud, seed, or fruit of an aromatic plant which grows in the tropics. Spices contain volatile oils which become stale if exposed to the air. With the exception of mustard seed, nearly all spices are imported in the United States.

Building up a spice repertoire is simple. One way is to purchase a small sample of an unfamiliar spice, examine it, taste it in the raw product, and try it in some food. Another approach is to wait until a recipe is found that requires an unfamiliar spice and then try it. One should not be afraid to try a new recipe with a never-before-used seasoning, but a taste-testing panel should be used before serving. At first one should not try for a striking flavor, but should use seasonings cautiously until one attains a subtle, not-too-pronounced flavor.

The main object in achieving well-seasoned foods is a blend of flavor accents in proper order. The first and last flavor impressions are important.

What is the trick to seasoning foods properly? What makes flavor leadership? The answer to both questions is *blended* flavor, which is not always easy to achieve; but any effort to give a product a right flavor is worthwhile.

Two or more flavors are needed for a blend, since most single flavors are not blended. Flavors occurring in nature are often blends.

There are a number of factors that should be considered when tasting a product to see whether it has been seasoned properly. A variety in flavors makes a food interesting. But the blending of spices or herbs is not accomplished if these ingredients are not compatible with the rest of the flavor notes in the product.

The order of appearance of flavor notes is a very important aspect of blending and seasoning foods. After-taste is a consequence of this aspect. The speed with which a specific flavor note appears depends on the nature of the spice or seasoning, on the quantity of the material used, and on the sensitivity of the person who is doing the tasting. The order of appearance of flavor notes is often a means of differentiating between a leader and a poor product. The first flavor notes appearing to a taster make an impression on him. This initial impression is often referred to as the impact of a food.

Flavors need to be understood and pampered. They are perishable and subject to deterioration in much the same way that the structure and appearance of foods deteriorate. Flavors need to be conserved or strengthened, or they may need to be increased, changed, or subdued, according to their role in food preparation. A high degree of understanding of these techniques is basic to all cooking and to all flavorful food.

To strike happy notes on the flavor "keyboard" the following do's and don'ts are suggested:

Do's

1. Use restraint; usually ¼ teaspoon of a dried herb is sufficient for four servings.
2. Crush leaf herbs.
3. Add well in advance to cold foods to allow blending of flavors.
4. Balance seasonings within a meal.

Don'ts

1. Use too many dried herbs; dried are more potent.
2. Use too many in one dish, unless tried previously.
3. Add dried herbs to cooked foods until the last hour of cooking.
4. Use spices or herbs in every dish or every course.

Herbs Naturale

Herbs are bushy plants, most of them, standing no more than a foot or so high; and their fragrance is almost unnoticeable. Perhaps because so little is known about herbs they seem almost foreign to many people.

If one walks through a sedate herb garden at sunset, the herbs may be easily identified: thyme, basil, marjoram, mint, tarragon. One may pick a leaf, crush it in the hand, and all its savor is released. Then one learns that which is plain or dull may actually be something flavorful and/or sweet.

To "cook with herbs" is to cook with care and affection, and to season food with respect is to honor its consumers.

As fascinating as herbs are in cookery, they are quite as fascinating to grow, and they are easy to handle. To grow herbs out-of-doors, the average family needs a patch of ground only about ten feet square. This patch will accommodate the following herbs: sweet basil, dill, burnet, chives, garlic, sweet marjoram, parsley, rosemary, spearmint, sage, and others.

Fresh herbs are more delectable than dried for many dishes—salads and omelets particularly.

Herbs should be taken freely as a gift from the green, breathing, natural world.

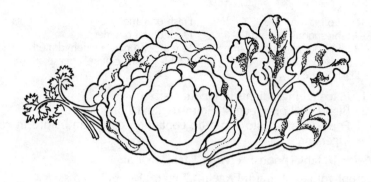

Nutritious, Beautiful Salads

People have been eating salad ingredients for centuries, but only in recent years have salads, as such, been widely served. There are almost limitless ways to combine mineral- and vitamin-rich foods in salad form. From a nutritional standpoint they are becoming more and more important in the daily menu. Salads are colorful and attractive.

A resourceful cook can vary the flavors of food as a composer varies his orchestral compositions. Colors and harmonies produce genuinely artistic as well as gastronomic pleasure.

The salad should complement the rest of the meal in color, texture, and combination. No matter how served, as part of a meal or as a separate course, salads provide more scope for the imagination than any other food preparation.

There are many principles to be considered in buying, storing, and cleaning foods used in salad preparation. Salad greens are of many varieties and in most cases form the foundation, or bed, for the salad. To insure crispness, all greens should be refrigerated at 38°–40° for at least two to four hours before using.

Lettuce comes in various forms and may be used in combination with other greens, vegetables, or fruits. Head lettuce is the most common, but other varieties include butterhead, leaf, bibb, romaine, and red lettuce. Endive comes in four varieties: endive, escarole, chicory, and French endive. Mustard greens, parsley, Chinese cabbage, and celery cabbage are also useful. Spinach and watercress are savory and often used in salad making.

Salad dressings are extremely important in enhancing flavor and appearance.

Creamy Ranch Dressing

½ cup mayonnaise
3 tablespoons buttermilk
3 tablespoons sour cream
¼ teaspoon salt
Dash garlic powder

Dash oregano, ground
Dash onion powder
½ teaspoon parsley, dehydrated
2 tablespoons cottage cheese

1. Place all ingredients in medium-size bowl.
2. Blend well on speed #1 in mixer for 15 minutes.
3. Pour dressing into a plastic container, cover, and store in refrigerator.

Yield: 16 tablespoons; *serving:* 1 tablespoon.

Carbohydrate, .4 gram; Protein, .7 gram; Fat, 6.3 grams.
Calories, 60 per serving.

Fruit and Oil Dressing

1 tablespoon oil
3 tablespoons orange juice or
   pineapple juice

1½ tablespoons papaya juice

1. Shake ingredients together in a jar and refrigerate.
2. Use on salads as desired.

Yield: ¼ cup; *serving:* 2 tablespoons.

Carbohydrate, 4.0 grams; Protein, .3 gram; Fat, 7.0 grams.
Calories, 79 per serving.

Low-Calorie Dressing

2 cups dry curd cottage
   cheese (packed)
1 cup yogurt
¼ teaspoon salt

1 cup buttermilk
2 tablespoons lemon herb seasoning
1 teaspoon lemon juice

1. Place all ingredients in mixing bowl.
2. Blend until smooth.

Yield: 4 cups or 64 tablespoons; *serving:* 1 tablespoon.

Carbohydrate, .6 gram; Protein, 1.3 grams; Fat, .8 gram.
Calories, 15 per serving.

Note: This is a basic recipe and may be varied by adding other seasonings to taste, or reserving the buttermilk to be added separately until the desired consistency is achieved.

Lemon Juice-Soy Mayonnaise

1 cup cold water (⅔ cup water)*
½ cup soy milk powder
1 cup oil (1¼ cups oil)*

½ teaspoon salt
Yellow food coloring (optional)
3 tablespoons or more lemon juice

Substitute measurements in parentheses.

Beater Method

1. Make a creamy paste of the soy milk powder and part of the water.
2. Add the oil gradually, beating thoroughly.
3. Add the remaining water as needed to thin the emulsion. It may be quite thin when the lemon juice is added, as the lemon juice causes the mixture to thicken.
4. Add the salt, yellow coloring, if desired, and lemon juice.
5. Beat together until smooth and creamy.

Liquefier Method

1. Place the water in the liquefier, add the soy milk powder. Whiz 1 minute.
2. Gradually add the oil while whizzing.
3. Add salt and yellow coloring, if desired.
4. Remove from the liquefier, and add the lemon juice.
5. Beat with a spoon until smooth and creamy.

Yield: 2½ cups; *serving:* ¼ cup.

Beater Method:
Carbohydrate, 1.6 grams; Protein, 2.4 grams; Fat, 28.5 grams. Calories, 273 per serving.

Liquefier Method:
Carbohydrate, 1.6 grams; Protein, 2.4 grams; Fat, 23.0 grams. Calories, 223 per serving.

Mock Roquefort Dressing

1 cup mayonnaise
1 cup low-fat yogurt
1 cup buttermilk

¼ teaspoon garlic salt
¼ teaspoon onion salt

1. Mix ingredients together.
2. Chill.

Yield: 3 cups; *servings:* 24 1-ounce

Carbohydrate, 1.1 grams; Protein, .9 gram; Fat, 6.9 grams. Calories, 68 per serving.

Russian Dressing—I

2 cups mayonnaise
⅔ cup chili sauce
1 egg, hard-boiled, diced

⅛ cup pickles, sweet, diced
¼ cup celery, diced

1. Mix above ingredients.
2. Blend until smooth.

Yield: 4 cups or 64 tablespoons.

Carbohydrate, 1.0 gram; Protein, .02 gram; Fat, 5.6 grams.
Calories, 54 per tablespoon.

Russian Dressing—II

1 cup cottage cheese
1 tablespoon lemon juice
¼ cup tomato juice

1 hard-boiled egg, finely chopped
1 small chopped onion
2 tablespoons parsley

1. Put the cottage cheese, onion, parsley, and lemon juice in an electric blender. Add ¼ cup tomato juice and blend until very smooth, adding more tomato juice if necessary.
2. Stir the egg into the dressing just before using.

Yield: 1 cup or 16 tablespoons.

Carbohydrate, .9 gram; Protein, 2.3 grams, Fat, .9 gram
Calories, 21 per tablespoon.

Tartar Sauce

2 cups mayonnaise
2 cups cream-of-tomato soup
  base
¼ cup parsley, chopped fine
1 tablespoon green onions,
  ground or chopped

¼ cup olives, pitted, chopped
½ cup dill pickle relish
4 eggs, hard-boiled or scrambled,
  chopped fine

1. Combine all ingredients.
2. Chill.

Yield: 6 cups or 96 tablespoons.

Carbohydrate, 1.0 gram; Protein, .4 gram; Fat, 4.0 grams.
Calories, 41 per tablespoon.

Yogurt Dressing

2 teaspoons lemon juice
1 tablespoon oil
½ cup plain low-fat yogurt
½ teaspoon paprika

Dash Tabasco
½ teaspoon salt
⅛ teaspoon garlic powder (optional)

1. Mix all ingredients together in a blender on medium speed for 5 seconds.
2. Chill.

Yield: ⅔ cup or 12 tablespoons

Carbohydrate, .5 gram; Protein, .3 gram; Fat, 1.3 grams.
Calories, 15 per tablespoon.

Zero-Salad Dressing

½ cup tomato juice
2 tablespoons lemon juice
1 tablespoon finely chopped onion

Salt to taste
Chopped parsley or green pepper (if desired)

1. Mix all ingredients well in jar with tightly fitted lid.
2. Shake before using.

Yield: ½ cup; servings: 4, 2 tablespoons each.

Carbohydrate, 2.1 grams; Protein, .4 gram; Fat, 1.0 gram.
Calories, 19 per serving.

Avocado and Grapefruit Salad

1 head romaine lettuce
1 avocado, pared and sliced
1 grapefruit, segments

½ cup cream, whipped
⅓ cup mayonnaise
½ teaspoon curry powder

1. Cut romaine in half, and arrange on plate.
2. Cover with alternate wedges of avocado and grapefruit.
3. Blend whipped cream with mayonnaise and curry powder.
4. Garnish and serve.

Yield: 8 servings.

Carbohydrate, 8.2 grams; Protein, 2.3 grams; Fat, 13.0 grams.
Calories, 159 per serving.

Peach Cardinal Salad

1 quart peach juice | Almond extract
¼ cup lemon juice | 6 large peach halves
½ cup cornstarch | 6 sprigs of parsley
1 or 2 tablespoons sugar | ¼ cup whipped cream

1. Divide juices in half. Heat one half to boiling.
2. Mix cold juices with cornstarch and sugar.
3. Add cold juice mixture to hot juice and boil again.
4. Remove from heat and add a little almond extract.
5. Cool.
6. If too thick, add more peach juice.
7. Place peach halves on tray with rounded side up.
8. Color the peach halves by using a pastry brush and applying the colored mixture.
9. Serve with star of whipped cream.
10. Garnish with parsley.

Note: Mayonnaise may be used in place of whipped cream.

Yield: 6 servings.

Carbohydrate, 34.7 grams; Protein, .4 gram; Fat, 1.9 gram.
Calories, 158 per serving.

Pineapple Boats

1 ripe pineapple | 2 cups fresh raspberries
1 ripe avocado | 2 bananas

1. Cut the pineapple in half crosswise.
2. Remove the inner core.
3. Save the shells.
4. Cube the pineapple and avocado; slice the strawberries and bananas.
5. Toss the fruits together.
6. Refill pineapple shells with the fruit mixture.
7. Serve for breakfast or a fruit dinner.

Yield: 6 servings; *serving:* 1 cup.

Carbohydrate, 19.6 grams; Protein, 1.4 grams; Fat, 6.3 grams.
Calories, 141 per serving.

Melon-Ball Fruit Cup

¼ cup (3 or 4) honeydew
  melon balls
½ cup (6 or 7) cantaloupe
  balls

⅛ cup blueberries
1 sprig of mint

1. Combine chilled melon and cantaloupe balls in serving cup. Sprinkle with the blueberries.
2. Garnish with mint sprig.

Yield: 1 serving; *serving:* 1 cup.

Carbohydrate, 12.4 grams; Protein, 1.0 gram; Fat, .2 gram.
Calories, 56 per serving.

Three-Fruit Salad

1 can peach pie filling
1 can pineapple chunks

1 can mandarin oranges
2 bananas, sliced

1. Combine all ingredients.
2. Let stand overnight.

Yield: 8 servings.

Carbohydrate, 52.0 grams; Protein, 2.0 grams; Fat, 5.0 grams.
Calories, 261 per serving.

Apricot-Cherry Mold

¾ cup lemon gelatin
1½ cups whole, peeled
  apricots, canned
½ cup juice from peeled
  apricots
½ cup plus 1 tablespoon
  apricot nectar

½ cup crushed pineapple, canned
½ cup cream cheese
3 tablespoons whipped topping
3 teaspoons red cherries
Several lettuce leaves

1. Mix juice from apricots and apricot nectar together. Heat to boiling.
2. Add gelatin and stir until well dissolved. Set aside.
3. Chop apricots, pineapple, and red cherries, and add to the gelatin mixture.
4. Add cream cheese and whipped topping. Mix until smooth.
5. Pour mixture into individual molds to set.
6. Unmold on plates garnished with lettuce leaves.
7. Arrange available fresh fruits around apricot mold.

Yield: 10 servings.

Carbohydrate, 24.0 grams; Protein, 2.9 grams; Fat, 5.7 grams.
Calories, 156 per serving.

Carrot-Pineapple Mold

1 3-ounce package orange or
  lemon gelatin
1 cup boiling water
½ cup mixed orange and
  pineapple juice
1 cup drained, crushed
  pineapple

1 cup raw, grated carrots
¼ cup chopped almonds
1 tablespoon minced green pepper

1. Dissolve the gelatin in boiling water.
2. Add fruit juice, and chill until slightly thickened.
3. Fold in remaining ingredients, and pour mixture into individual
   molds or a 1-quart mold.

Yield: 6 servings.

Carbohydrate, 31.5 grams; Protein, 2.8 grams; Fat, 3.2 grams.
Calories, 166 per serving.

Raspberry-Applesauce Mold

⅔ cup raspberry Jello
1 cup plus 1 tablespoon
  boiling water
1 cup applesauce
¾ cup frozen raspberries,
  thawed

⅔ cup sour cream
¼ cup miniature marshmallows
Several lettuce leaves

1. Dissolve Jello in boiling water.
2. Chill Jello until slightly thickened.
3. Add applesauce and thawed raspberries.
4. Pour mixture into Jello mold and chill until firm (overnight).
5. To unmold: dip mold in hot water for few seconds.
6. Place a few lettuce leaves on top of mold.
7. Place a platter over lettuce leaves, then turn entire contents
   upside down.
8. Combine sour cream and marshmallows.
9. Top Jello mold with sour cream/marshmallow mixture.

Yield: 10 servings.

Carbohydrate, 24.0 grams; Protein, 3.0 grams; Fat, 3.0 grams.
Calories, 135 per serving.

Cranberry-Orange Salad

1 3-ounce package lemon
  gelatin
1 cup boiling water
1 cup orange juice

1 16-ounce jar cranberry-orange relish
1 unpeeled apple, chopped
½ cup pecans, chopped

1. Dissolve gelatin in boiling water.
2. Add orange juice and let stand until almost jelled.
3. Combine cranberry-orange relish, chopped apple, and pecans;
   fold into the almost-jelled mixture.
4. Pour mixture into a 1-quart mold.
5. Chill until firm.

Yield: 10 small servings.

Carbohydrate, 38.3 grams; Protein, 1.7 grams; Fat, 4.5 grams.
Calories, 201 per serving.

Sunshine Mold

1½ cups crushed pineapple,
  canned
3¾ cups boiling water
1 large package orange
  gelatin

½ cup carrots, shredded
1 cup mayonnaise
Lettuce leaves

1. Drain pineapple thoroughly for ½ to 1 hour.
2. Dissolve gelatin in boiling water and stir well. Let set until
   thickened.
3. Add pineapple, mayonnaise, and shredded carrots. Mix well.
4. Pour mixture into individual molds.
5. Refrigerate to set.
6. Unmold gelatin onto lettuce-garnished salad plates.

Yield: 10 servings.

Carbohydrate, 9.7 grams; Protein, .6 gram; Fat, 17.0 grams.
Calories, 190 per serving.

Tomato Aspic Mold

1¾ cups tomato juice
½ teaspoon salt
1 bay leaf
½ teaspoon paprika
1 teaspoon lemon juice
1 tablespoon grated onions

1 tablespoon unflavored gelatin (1 envelope)
¼ cup cold water
½ cup celery, chopped
2 tablespoons green onions, chopped
2 tablespoons parsley, finely chopped

1. Heat together tomato juice, salt, and bay leaf.
2. Remove from heat, take out bay leaf, and add paprika, lemon juice, and grated onions.
3. Soften gelatin in the cold water and combine with the hot tomato juice mixture.
4. Stir until dissolved. Cool.
5. Add chopped vegetables.
6. Pour into 6 individual molds and refrigerate until set.

Yield: 6 servings.

Carbohydrate, 4.0 grams; Protein, 2.0 grams; Fat, trace.
Calories, 24.0 per serving.

Cabbage and Apple Slaw

2 medium, red, eating apples
¼ cup pineapple juice

2 cups cabbage, finely shredded
¾ cup Sweet-and-Sour Dressing

1. Wash and core apples.
2. Chop in chopper.
3. Place chopped apples in pineapple juice and mix well.
4. Drain apples and mix with shredded cabbage and dressing.

Sweet-and-Sour Dressing

⅔ cup mayonnaise
2 teaspoons sugar

3 tablespoons lemon juice

1. Combine all ingredients.
2. Blend well.
3. Refrigerate before serving.

Yield: 10 servings.

Carbohydrate, 9.9 grams; Protein, .8 gram; Fat, 11.0 grams.
Calories, 140 per serving.

California Slaw Salad

1¼ cups pineapple chunks
2 cups cabbage, finely
   shredded
1¼ cups miniature
   marshmallows

1½ cups Sour Cream Dressing
½ cup mandarin oranges
10 red cherry halves

1. Drain pineapple thoroughly for ½ to 1 hour.
2. Combine cabbage, pineapple, mandarin oranges, and marsh-mallows with sour cream dressing.
3. Portion salad into servings.
4. Garnish each salad with a red cherry half.

Sour Cream Dressing I

1 cup sour cream
½ cup mayonnaise
1 teaspoon sugar

1 tablespoon lemon juice
¼ teaspoon salt

1. Combine all ingredients.
2. Blend with an electric mixer.

Yield: 10 servings.

Carbohydrate, 16.0 grams; Protein, 1.8 grams; Fat, 10.0 grams.
Calories, 159 per serving.

Carrot-Pineapple Salad

1 cup pineapple, crushed
1½ pounds carrots, shredded

½ teaspoon salt
1 cup Sour Cream Dressing

1. Combine pineapple, carrots, salt, and Sour Cream Dressing, and mix well.
2. Garnish plates with lettuce.
3. Place ½ cup carrot-pineapple mixture on each garnished plate.

Sour Cream Dressing II

½ cup sour cream
2 tablespoons mayonnaise
½ teaspoon sugar

1 teaspoon lemon juice
¼ teaspoon salt

1. Mix all ingredients.
2. Blend with an electric mixer.

Yield: 10 servings.

Carbohydrate, 12.0 grams; Protein, 1.5 grams; Fat, 7.0 grams.
Calories, 115 per serving.

Carrot-Coconut Salad

5 cups shredded carrots
4 teaspoons shredded
coconut
½ teaspoon salt

¾ cup Sweet-and-Sour Dressing (see p. 156)
Several lettuce leaves
10 black olives, pitted

1. Combine carrots, coconut, salt, and Sweet-and-Sour Dressing in bowl, and mix thoroughly.
2. Line salad plates with lettuce leaves.
3. Place ½ cup of carrot mixture on each garnished dish.
4. Garnish each salad with an olive.

Yield: 10 servings.

Carbohydrate, 9.0 grams; Protein, 1.2 grams; Fat, 6.0 grams.
Calories, 95 per serving.

Carrot-Pineapple-Raisin Salad

1½ cups pineapple, crushed
1½ pounds carrots, shredded
⅔ cup raisins
½ cup Sour Cream Dressing
(see p. 157)

10 red cherry halves
3 tablespoons shredded coconut
Lettuce leaves

1. Garnish salad plates with lettuce.
2. Drain pineapple thoroughly for ½ to 1 hour, then add to carrots.
3. Place raisins in hot water and let stand about 5 minutes.
4. Mix carrots, pineapple, and raisins with Sour Cream Dressing.
5. Place ½ cup portion onto garnished plates.
6. Garnish with a red cherry half and a sprinkle of coconut.

Yield: 10 servings.

Carbohydrate, 22.0 grams; Protein, 1.6 grams; Fat, 5.8 grams.
Calories, 146 per serving.

Carrot-Raisin Salad

5 cups shredded carrots
¾ cup raisins
1¼ cups mayonnaise

1 tablespoon plus ½ teaspoon
pineapple juice
2 tablespoons sugar
Lettuce leaves

1. Combine shredded carrots, raisins, mayonnaise, pineapple juice, and sugar in bowl, and mix well.
2. Place ½ cup carrot mixture on each lettuce-garnished dish.

Yield: 10 servings.

Carbohydrate, 15.0 grams; Protein, 1.2 grams; Fat, 21.0 grams.
Calories, 254 per serving.

Cauliflower Salad

1 medium cauliflower	½ cup mayonnaise
1 carrot	Salt to taste
2 medium tomatoes	Lettuce leaves

1. Wash, trim, and dry cauliflower.
2. Put carrot through fine grater.
3. Dice tomatoes.
4. Mix carrot, tomatoes, salt, and mayonnaise.
5. Grate cauliflower on large side of grater (or chop coarsely with knife).
6. Toss cauliflower lightly with other vegetables.
7. Serve on lettuce leaves.

Yield: 6 servings; *serving:* ½ cup.

Carbohydrate, 6.5 grams; Protein, 2.2 grams; Fat, 13.8 grams. Calories, 159 per serving.

Cauliflower and Cheese Salad

1 medium head cauliflower	½ cup Cheddar cheese, shredded
⅓ cup mayonnaise	⅓ cup black olives, pitted
⅓ cup sour cream	Several lettuce leaves

1. Cook cauliflower 7 minutes. Chill.
2. Blend mayonnaise and sour cream.
3. Garnish salad plates with lettuce leaves.
4. Assemble salads by placing cauliflower on each plate.
5. Top with dressing and sprinkle with Cheddar cheese.
6. Garnish with olives.

Yield: 6 servings.

Carbohydrate, 1.2 grams; Protein, 3.0 grams; Fat, 16.0 grams. Calories, 164 per serving.

Celery-Seed Coleslaw

3 cups finely shredded cabbage	1 tablespoon chopped pimento
3 tablespoons oil	2 tablespoons sugar
⅓ cup lemon juice, warmed	½ teaspoon salt
1 tablespoon finely-chopped onion	½ teaspoon celery seeds

1. In a large bowl toss the shredded cabbage, oil, and warm lemon juice.
2. Add the remaining ingredients and toss again.
3. Cover and refrigerate until serving time.

Yield: 6 servings.

Carbohydrate, 8.0 grams; Protein, .6 gram; Fat, 7.0 grams. Calories, 97 per serving.

Coleslaw-Ribbon Salad

3¼ cups cabbage, finely shredded
¼ cup red cabbage, finely shredded

1½ cups Coleslaw Dressing

1. Place cabbage and dressing in bowl.
2. Mix well.

Coleslaw Dressing

½ cup mayonnaise
1 cup Creamy Ranch Dressing
(see p. 148)
¾ teaspoon celery seed

Dash onion powder
½ teaspoon salt
¾ tablespoon lemon juice

Yield: 10 servings.

Carbohydrate, 6.7 grams; Protein, 2.2 grams; Fat, 16.0 grams.
Calories, 181 per serving.

Coleslaw Tangy Salad

4½ cups cabbage, finely shredded
⅓ cup green peppers, finely sliced
⅓ cup red onions, finely sliced

2 tablespoons lemon juice
2 tablespoons sugar
¼ teaspoon salt
¼ cup sour cream
¾ cup mayonnaise

1. Place vegetables in large bowl. Set aside.
2. Combine lemon juice, sugar, salt, sour cream, and mayonnaise.
3. Blend until smooth.
4. Toss vegetables lightly with dressing.

Yield: 10 servings.

Carbohydrate, 6.0 grams; Protein, 1.0 gram; Fat, 14.0 grams.
Calories, 152 per serving.

Chef's Salad

1 head iceberg lettuce
½ cup celery, sliced
⅓ cup radishes, thinly sliced
⅓ cup cucumbers, unpeeled, sliced
4 slices American cheese cut in strips

½ cup "209" turkey-flavor soyameat slices, cut into ¼ inch strips (see p. 174)
1 small avocado
1 teaspoon lemon juice
1 cup water

1. Place lettuce, celery, radishes, and cucumbers in large bowl and toss lightly.
2. Combine water and lemon juice.
3. Peel avocado, slice, and dip in lemon juice solution.
4. Place 1 cup of salad into each salad bowl.
5. Garnish each salad with 3 cheese strips, 3 "209" turkey-flavor strips, and 1 avocado wedge.

Yield: 10 servings.

Carbohydrate, 3.7 grams; Protein, 4.1 grams; Fat, 6.3 grams.
Calories, 88 per serving.

Chef's Spinach Salad

1 pound raw spinach
⅔ cup cooked chick peas
½ cup sliced mushrooms
½ cup sliced beets
8 ounces farmer's or ricotta cheese (made from partially skimmed milk)

⅓ cup pumpkin or sunflower seeds
Juice of one lemon
2 tablespoons oil

1. Wash spinach and break into bite-size pieces.
2. Toss chick peas, mushrooms, beets, and crumbled farmer's cheese with spinach.
3. Just before serving, sprinkle in seeds, and add the lemon juice and oil as dressing.

Yield: 10 servings.

Carbohydrate, 13.0 grams; Protein, 8.0 grams; Fat, 6.0 grams.
Calories, 138 per serving.

Chick-Pea Platter

2 cans (1 pound each) chick-
  peas, drained, or 1 cup
  dried chick-peas, soaked,
  cooked, and drained
⅓ cup chopped scallions
2 tablespoons chopped
  parsley

¼ cup oil
2 tablespoons lemon juice
½ teaspoon salt
Salad greens

1. Combine the chick-peas, scallions, and parsley.
2. Blend together the oil, lemon juice, and salt, and pour over the vegetables.
3. Toss lightly.
4. Chill well, at least one hour, tossing twice during chilling.
5. Serve on bed of crisp salad greens.

Yield: 10 servings.

Carbohydrate, 12.0 grams; Protein, 4.0 grams; Fat, 7.0 grams.
Calories, 127 per serving.

"Chicken"-Vegetable Salad

2 cups Soyameat, chicken-
  like flavor, diced (see p. 174)
½ cucumber, peeled and
  diced
½ cup diced celery
½ cup water chestnuts,
  drained and sliced

¼ cup diced green pepper
¼ cup sliced scallions
¼ cup mayonnaise
6 lettuce cups
2 tablespoons capers
Paprika

1. Toss the first 6 ingredients with mayonnaise.
2. Serve in lettuce cups, garnish with capers and paprika.

Yield: 6 servings.

Carbohydrate, 7.0 grams; Protein, 7.0 grams; Fat, 14.0 grams.
Calories, 182 per serving.

Chilled Tomato-Accordion Salad

5 medium tomatoes
¾ cup Soyameat, chicken-
like flavor, diced (ground)
(see p. 174)
2 tablespoons celery, finely
chopped
1 tablespoon sweet pickle
relish

⅔ cup mayonnaise
⅜ teaspoon curry powder
¼ teaspoon salt
10 black olives, pitted

1. Cut tomatoes in half and place halves on cut side. Without cutting to the bottom, make 3 slices (accordion).
2. Combine Soyameat, celery, sweet pickle relish, mayonnaise, curry powder, and salt.
3. Use pastry tube to place mixture between tomato slices.
4. Garnish with black olives.

Yield: 10 servings.

Carbohydrate, 5.0 grams; Protein, 3.0 grams; Fat, 11.0 grams.
Calories, 129 per serving.

Corn Salad

1 cup cooked corn kernels,
cut from the cob
1½ cups cottage cheese,
well-drained
1 tablespoon chopped green
pepper

1 tablespoon chopped parsley
Salt to taste

1. Toss all ingredients together.
2. Store in a covered container in the refrigerator until serving time.

Yield: 4 servings.

Carbohydrate, 10.0 grams; Protein, 12.0 grams; Fat, 3.5 grams.
Calories, 116 per serving.

Cucumber and Onion Salad

1 pound cucumbers, thinly
sliced
1 small onion, cut into thin
rings
½ cup sour cream

½ teaspoon salt
1 teaspoon lemon juice
¾ teaspoon sugar

1. Peel cucumbers, score with a fork, then slice thin.
2. Slice onions thin.
3. Pour sour cream over cucumbers and mix lightly.

Yield: 10 servings.

Carbohydrate, 3.4 grams; Protein, 1.0 gram; Fat, 1.4 grams.
Calories, 28 per serving.

Full-Meal Salad

1 clove garlic, crushed
½ cup diced celery
½ cup sliced onions
¼ cup chopped green
  scallions
2 apples, finely chopped
1½ cups chopped raw
  broccoli flowerets
4 radishes, sliced
½ cup diced green pepper
½ cup tangerine sections
1 cup mixed nuts
1 cup diced cheese
1 head romaine lettuce, core, chopped
  and leaves shredded
The hard core of one large cabbage,
  chopped
1 cup raisins
1½ cups whole-wheat or rye-bread
  toast cubes
2 tablespoons margarine
1½ cups mayonnaise

1. Rub a salad bowl with the clove of garlic.
2. Combine all the ingredients except the toast cubes, margarine,
   and mayonnaise in the bowl, and mix well.
3. Add enough of the mayonnaise to moisten the salad. Toss well.
4. Toss toast cubes in melted butter.
5. Sprinkle salad with the toast cubes.

Yield: 16 servings.

Carbohydrate, 19.0 grams; Protein, 6.0 grams; Fat, 23.0 grams.
Calories, 302 per serving.

Lettuce Salad

½ clove garlic
1 head lettuce
2 tablespoons parsley,
  chopped
1 tablespoon scallions,
  chopped
2 tablespoons onion, finely
  chopped
1 cup watercress sprigs
1 tablespoon lemon juice
½ tablespoon sesame paste
⅛ teaspoon tarragon
Salt to taste

1. Rub salad bowl with the garlic clove.
2. Add the lettuce, parsley, scallions, onion, and watercress.
3. Beat together lemon juice and sesame paste.
4. Add tarragon and salt.
5. Pour over greens.
6. Toss with wooden spoon and fork.

Note: Dandelion leaves, 1 quart, may be substituted for the lettuce.
Pick the dandelion greens before the flowers blossom.

Yield: 4 servings; *serving:* 1 cup.

Carbohydrate, 5.6 grams; Protein, 2.0 grams; Fat, 3.5 grams.
Calories, 62 per serving.

Grated Salad

3 cups grated cabbage
2 cups grated carrots
½ cup finely peeled,
  chopped broccoli
⅓ cup sesame seeds
1 diced tomato

½ cup chopped cucumber
¼ cup chopped green pepper
¼ cup chopped celery
½ avocado, diced, dipped in lemon
  juice

1. In a large salad bowl combine the cabbage, carrots, broccoli, and sesame seeds.
2. Use the tomato, avocado, cucumber, green pepper, and celery to garnish the salad in an attractive platter.
3. At the table, toss the salad with dressing.

Yield: 8 servings; *serving:* 1 cup.

Carbohydrate, 8.6 grams; Protein, 2.8 grams; Fat, 6.3 grams.
Calories, 102 per serving.

Gado-Gado Salad

"Indonesian"

½ head lettuce
1 tomato, diced
½ cup water chestnuts
½ cup chopped cabbage

1 cup bean sprouts
1 cup sliced cooked potatoes
1 cup cooked beans
1 cup fried tofu (bean curd)

1. Line platter with lettuce leaves.
2. Arrange remaining ingredients in the order listed.
3. Cover with Peanut Butter Sauce.

Peanut Butter Sauce

1 small onion, minced
1 medium clove garlic,
  minced
Salt to taste or ½ teaspoon
1 tablespoon sugar
⅓ cup peanut butter, smooth
  or crunchy

1 cup water
1 tablespoon lemon juice
1 teaspoon soy sauce
1 teaspoon catsup

1. Sauté onion and garlic until tender and light brown.
2. Add salt and sugar.
3. Add the peanut butter, then gradually add the water until consistency of soft butter.
4. Add the lemon juice, soy sauce, and catsup.

Yield: 4 servings.

Salad:

Carbohydrate, 19.0 grams; Protein,
8.5 grams; Fat, 4.0 grams.
Calories, 146 per serving.

Sauce:

Carbohydrate, 8.0 grams; Protein,
5.5 grams; Fat, 10.0 grams.
Calories, 144 per serving.

Luncheon Salad

1 medium zucchini or 1
  medium cucumber
4 stalks celery with leaves
¼ green pepper
1 carrot
5 sprigs parsley

2 tomatoes
2 green onions with tops
1 cup cooked garbanzos or other
  cooked beans
4 lettuce cups

1. Quarter the zucchini or cucumber lengthwise and slice thin.
2. Remove the strings from the celery, and slice the stalk, including the leaves, crosswise.
3. Chop the parsley and the green pepper.
4. Shred the carrot.
5. Peel the tomatoes and cut into wedges.
6. Slice the onions, using much of the green part.
7. Add the cooked garbanzos or beans, and toss lightly together with lemon juice, or creamy French dressing.
8. Pile lightly into the lettuce cups.

Note: May use radish roses for garnish.

Yield: 4 servings.

Carbohydrate, 22.0 grams; Protein, 6.0 grams; Fat, 3.0 grams.
Calories, 139 per serving.

Romaine and Radish Salad

4 cups romaine leaves
8 radishes, quartered
1 scallion, chopped
¼ cup walnut pieces
½ cored apple, unpeeled and
  diced

4 dates, chopped
1 tablespoon raisins
2 tablespoons fresh dill weed
2 tablespoons chopped parsley

1. Combine all ingredients in a wooden bowl.
2. Mix together the yogurt and other dressing ingredients as listed in recipe below.
3. Pour over the salad and toss the mixture.

Dressing

⅓ cup yogurt
1 tablespoon lemon juice

1 tablespoon honey
1 tablespoon sesame seeds, toasted

Yield: 10 servings.

Carbohydrate, 9.6 grams; Protein, 1.5 grams; Fat, 3.1 grams.
Calories, 73 per serving.

Mediterranean Cucumber Salad

2 small, firm cucumbers
1 cup yogurt
3 tablespoons raisins
¼ cup chopped walnuts

1 small onion, finely chopped
Salt to taste
1 tablespoon finely chopped fresh mint leaves

1. Peel cucumbers, slice lengthwise.
2. Dice cucumbers and place in a bowl.
3. Add remaining ingredients and mix well.
4. Chill and serve very cold.

Yield: 4 servings.

Carbohydrate, 14.0 grams; Protein, 4.5 grams; Fat, 7.0 grams.
Calories, 137 per serving.

Mock Tuna Fish Salad

3 cups Meatless Chicken slices (frozen) (see p. 174)
1 7-ounce can Tartex, plain (see p. 174)
1 stalk celery, finely chopped

1 tablespoon onion, finely chopped
½ cup mayonnaise
½ to 1 teaspoon paprika

1. Grind Meatless Chicken slices, celery, and onion together.
2. Combine all ingredients.
3. Mix well.

Note: This salad may be used also as a sandwich filling.

Carbohydrate, 6.0 grams; Protein, 18.0 grams; Fat, 15.0 grams.
Calories, 230 per serving.

Peas-Peanut Salad

2 cups tender green peas (frozen or fresh)
1 cup thinly diced celery
½ cup Spanish peanuts (or 1 cup cubed Nuteena, see p. 174)

1 pimento, diced
½ cup soy or regular mayonnaise
1 cup toasted croutons

1. Add peas to small amount of salted boiling water; cook 2 minutes; drain, cool, and chill.
2. Combine all ingredients except croutons.
3. Add croutons just before serving.
4. Toss lightly.

Yield: 8 servings.

Carbohydrate, 10.7 grams; Protein, 3.0 grams; Fat, 18.2 grams.
Calories, 219 per serving.

Special Dinner Salad

2 cups shredded romaine
2 cups shredded spinach
  leaves
1 tablespoon safflower oil
¼ cup imitation bacon bits
  (see p. 174)
1 hard-cooked egg, grated
4 thin carrot sticks

4 ripe olives
1 tomato, cut into wedges
1 tablespoon chopped fresh basil
1 tablespoon fresh dill weed
Lemon juice to taste

1. Combine the romaine and spinach in a salad bowl.
2. Add the oil and toss the mixture until all the leaves glisten.
3. Add imitation bacon bits, egg, carrot sticks, olives, tomato, basil, and dill weed.
4. Toss the mixture again.
5. Add lemon juice and salt.

Yield: 6 servings.

Carbohydrate, 4.0 grams; Protein, 4.0 grams; Fat, 4.0 grams.
Calories, 68 per serving.

Spinach-Grapefruit Salad

1 bunch raw spinach (about
  12 ounces as purchased)
2 grapefruit, peeled,
  sectioned
2 tomatoes, cut in bite-size
  pieces

1 tablespoon toasted sesame seeds
¼ cup sesame oil
2 tablespoons lemon juice

1. Remove stems from spinach and wash thoroughly; dry and break into bite-size pieces.
2. Chill until serving time.
3. Combine spinach, grapefruit sections, and tomato pieces.
4. Combine sesame seeds, oil, and lemon juice; shake well.
5. Pour over spinach mixture and toss lightly.

Yield: 6 servings.

Carbohydrate, 13.0 grams; Protein, 3.0 grams; Fat, 10.0 grams.
Calories, 154 per serving.

Stuffed-Tomato Salad

10 tomatoes, medium size
9 ounces cream cheese or
cottage cheese
2 small green onions, finely
chopped
10 radishes, finely chopped

1 small stalk celery, finely chopped
4 sprigs of watercress, finely chopped
Pinch of salt

1. Dip tomatoes, a few at a time, in boiling water.
2. Plunge into cold water.
3. Peel tomatoes; core and chill.
4. Prepare filling of chopped vegetables, cream cheese, and salt.
5. Cream until smooth.
6. Cut tomatoes in 6ths, only ⅔ of the way down.
7. Spread carefully, do not break.
8. Fill tomatoes with filling.

Yield: 10 servings; *serving:* 1 tomato.

Carbohydrate, 8.6 grams; Protein, 8.8 grams; Fat, 9.1 grams.
Calories, 152 per serving.

Tabouli Salad

(Zesty Lebanese Salad)

¼ cup garbanzos, cooked
and drained (optional)
1¼ cups bulgur wheat, raw
4 cups boiling water
1½ cups minced parsley
¾ cup mint, minced (if not
available, substitute more
parsley)
3 medium tomatoes, chopped

¾ cup lemon juice
¼ cup olive oil
½ teaspoon salt
Raw grape, lettuce, or cabbage leaves
¾ cup minced scallions

1. Pour the boiling water over the bulgur wheat and let stand about
2 hours until the wheat is light and fluffy.
2. Drain excess water and shake wheat in a strainer or press with
hands to remove as much water as possible.
3. Mix the bulgur wheat, cooked beans, if used, and remaining
ingredients.
4. Chill for at least 1 hour.
5. Serve on raw leaves.

Yield: 12 servings.

Carbohydrate, 17.6 grams; Protein, 2.8 grams; Fat, 5.1 grams.
Calories, 127 per serving.

Tostada Salad

1 cup kidney beans, canned
2 tablespoons onion, diced
2 tablespoons black olives, chopped
½ cup Cheddar Cheese, shredded
1 small head iceberg lettuce

½ cup tomatoes, diced
½ cup Ranch Dressing
½ cup avocado
6½-ounce corn chips (large package)

1. Drain kidney beans well.
2. Peel and mash avocado.
3. Combine kidney beans, onions, olives, cheese, lettuce, tomatoes, and mashed avocado.
4. Add Ranch Dressing, then toss mixture lightly.
5. Garnish salad plates with green lettuce.
6. Place salad serving on garnished plate.
7. Place corn chips on top of salad.

Ranch Dressing

2 tablespoons mayonnaise
1 tablespoon buttermilk
2 tablespoons sour cream
Dash salt

Dash garlic powder
Dash ground oregano
¼ teaspoon parsley, dehydrated
1½ teaspoons cottage cheese

1. Place all ingredients in medium bowl.
2. Blend well on speed #1 in mixer. Mix for 15 seconds.
3. Pour dressing into plastic container, cover, and store in refrigerator.

Yield: 10 servings.

Carbohydrate, 14.0 grams; Protein, 5.0 grams; Fat, 15.0 grams.
Calories, 213 per serving.

Tofu Salad Deluxe

1 cup tofu, steamed and
  diced
1 cup grated carrots or diced
  apples
½ cup raisins
½ cup walnut meats, coarsely
  chopped
2 teaspoons sugar
2 tablespoons sesame seeds
4 lettuce leaves

1. Combine all ingredients, and mix well.
2. If desired, serve mixture in mounds on lettuce leaves.

Yield: 4 servings.

Salad with Carrots:
Carbohydrate, 23.0 grams; Protein,
11.0 grams; Fat, 14.0 grams.
Calories, 262 per serving.

Salad with Apples:
Carbohydrate, 25.0 grams; Protein,
9.0 grams; Fat, 14.0 grams.
Calories, 262 per serving.

Zucchini Salad

3 small, young zucchini
3 scallions, finely chopped
2 tablespoons dill weed, fresh
1 tablespoon parsley,
  chopped
¼ teaspoon oregano
1 cup plain yogurt
1 tablespoon lemon juice
1 teaspoon honey

1. Wash zucchini, then dice it very fine.
2. Place zucchini in salad bowl with scallions, dill, parsley, and oregano.
3. Combine yogurt, lemon juice, and honey, then pour over zucchini mixture.
4. Toss well.
5. Refrigerate 30 minutes or longer before serving.

Yield: 5 servings; *serving:* ½ cup.

Carbohydrate, 6.5 grams; Protein, 2.9 grams; Fat, 1.0 gram.
Calories, 47 per serving.

About Main Dishes . . .

The following section features outstanding recipes for vegetarian main dishes which have long been enjoyed by visitors and patients alike at Glendale Adventist Medical Center in Southern California.

These first several pages offer important information about special protein ingredients as well as recipes for the delicious sauces and gravies often used as accompaniments.

Page 173: A discussion about cheeses.

Page 174: Brief descriptions of vegetarian meat-like products available in most markets and health food stores—as well as special seasonings to impart meat-like flavors.

Page 175: Sauces and gravies. (Other sauces designed for specific recipes appear with those recipes.)

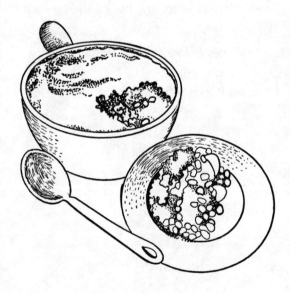

The Use of Cheese

This book contains recipes using some cheeses. Cheese is an excellent source of protein, and also may be used for flavor and garnish. Whatever its function, one should be aware of the various cheeses available and their composition.

Some cheeses are more easily digested than others, and, because the best quality is desired as well as the most nutritious, the strong, sharp cheeses should be avoided. The most wholesome are the unripened cheeses such as cottage cheese, cream cheese, and American cheese. The butterfat is high in cream cheese (20–40%), and for this reason it should be used sparingly. Whatever the cheese, its source should be clean, and all products should be pasteurized.

In the processing of ripening cheeses such as Cheddar, Limburger, and Swiss, a bacterium, lactobacillus, is used for fermentation. The activity of the bacteria slowly ferments milk sugar and protein. The resulting decomposition products provide the textures and flavors of ripened cheeses.

In the preparation of cheese, changes in the composition of the milk occur. First, the curd is separated from the whey. The degree of this concentration depends on the type of cheese being made, on the type of milk being used, and on the manner of coagulation. The protein in cheese also depends on the method of coagulation. The coagulation may be done by adding a starter culture, such as the milk-coagulating enzyme rennet, and by controlling the cooking temperatures.

Today there are many low-fat and low-salt cheeses available. Those with the lowest fat content should be selected.

In summary, cheeses are not the most easily digested foods, and the yellow cheeses should be used sparingly because of their high concentration of protein and fat. Cream cheese is the most easily digested, but contains much fat that makes it high in calories. The most easily digested cheeses are cottage cheese, pot cheese, cream cheese, Neufchâtel, and ricotta. For health reasons, these cheeses may be readily adapted in many of the recipes that require cheese. Cottage cheese, a source of high quality protein, is relatively low in calories, and makes a significant contribution to the daily calcium requirement.

Vegetable Protein Alternates (Analogues)

Meat alternates, or analogues, are used in some of the recipes in this book. They may be beef-like, chicken-like, fish-like, ham-like, sausage-like, or turkey-like. The products come canned, frozen, or dehydrated, and may incorporate soybean, wheat, or nut protein.

Several companies make products that are somewhat similar. Most of those used in these recipes are products of Loma Linda Foods, 11503 Pierce St., Riverside, CA 92515; and Worthington Foods, Worthington, OH 43085.

Meat analogues are available in many stores including health food stores, or one may write the companies asking for outlets nearby. Many products are offered in addition to those in these recipes.

Beef-like

Canned
 Dinner Cuts
 Non-Meat Balls
 Nuteena
 Prime Stakes
 Proteena
 Soyameat, slices
 Tastee Cuts
 Vege-Burger
 Vegetable Steaks

Frozen
 Corned "Beef" Style Luncheon
  Slices, or roll
 Prime, slices or roll

Dehydrated
 GranBurger, textured vegetable
  protein

Seasonings and Other Special Products

 Marmite, Vegex, Savorex, yeast
  extract products
 BacoChips, imitation bacon bits
 Tartex, paté-like spread
 Bakon Yeast, smoked flavoring
 Beef-like, chicken-like, etc.,
  seasonings, available in vari-
  ous brands and forms
 Gravy-Quik, a gravy mix

Chicken-like

Canned
 FriChik
 Soyameat, slices
 Tender Bits

Frozen
 Chic-ketts
 Meatless Chicken, roll or slices
 White Chix, slices

Fish-like

Canned
 Vegetable Skallops

Turkey-like

Canned
 "209," slices

Ham-like

Frozen
 Wham

Sausage-like

Canned
 Veja-Links

Frozen
 Saucettes
 RX

Sauces and Gravies

Medium White Sauce

2½ tablespoons margarine
3 tablespoons all-purpose
  flour

2 cups non-fat milk
½ teaspoon salt

1. Melt margarine.
2. Add flour and mix until smooth.
3. Heat milk and add to flour and margarine mixture.
4. Stir with a wire whip. Add salt.
5. Cook until thickened.

Yield: 2 cups; *serving:* ¼ cup.

Carbohydrate, 5.8 grams; Protein, 2.8 grams; Fat, 3.8 grams.
Calories, 66 per serving.

Thin White Sauce, Thick White Sauce

For a thin white sauce, use 2 tablespoons margarine and 2 tablespoons flour. For a thick white sauce, use 3 tablespoons margarine and 4 tablespoons flour.

Brown Gravy

4 tablespoons margarine
4 tablespoons all-purpose
  flour
2 tablespoons beef-flavor
  seasoning (see p. 174)

½ teaspoon onion salt
2 cups hot water

1. Combine flour, beef-flavor seasoning, and onion salt.
2. Add to margarine and cook to golden brown, stirring frequently to prevent burning.
3. Add water and bring to a boil. Simmer slowly for 5 to 10 minutes. More or less water may be used depending on desired consistency.

Yield: 2 cups; *serving:* ¼ cup.

Carbohydrate, 2.4 grams; Protein, 1.6 grams; Fat, 3.2 grams.
Calories, 44 per serving.

Mushroom Gravy

¼ cup mushrooms
1 tablespoon onion, minced

1 tablespoon margarine
2 cups Medium White Sauce

1. Add mushrooms, minced onions, and margarine to Medium White Sauce.
2. Heat thoroughly before serving.

Yield: 2 cups; *serving:* ¼ cup.

Carbohydrate, 7.0 grams; Protein, 3.7 grams; Fat, 8.3 grams.
Calories, 118 per serving.

Vegetarian Main Dishes

Baked Italian Loaf

1½ pounds Prime Stakes (see p. 174)
1 cup chopped onions, braised
4 eggs
1¼ cups bread crumbs
2 cups half-and-half cream
1 teaspoon sage
½ cup chopped parsley
½ cup Parmesan cheese
1 cup tomato paste

1. Grind Prime Stakes coarsely.
2. Mix all ingredients except cheese and tomato paste.
3. Pour mixture into oiled pan.
4. Spread tomato paste and Parmesan cheese on loaf.
5. Cover loaf with another pan and bake at 300°F for 1½ hours.

Yield: 10 servings.

Carbohydrate, 10.2 grams; Protein, 15.5 grams; Fat, 12.6 grams.
Calories, 216 per serving.

Bean-Walnut Patties

1 cup brown beans, cooked and mashed
½ cup walnuts
1 onion
2 tablespoons flour
1 teaspoon Italian seasoning
¼ cup bean broth or warm water
1 egg, beaten
1 teaspoon salt

1. Finely chop the walnuts.
2. Cut onion finely and sauté lightly in oil.
3. Add flour and allow to heat.
4. Add broth or warm water, and stir to smooth paste.
5. Finally, add egg, beans, walnuts, seasoning, and salt.
6. Mix well, form into patties, and roll in flour.
7. Cook in a greased pan until brown and firm.
8. Serve hot with tomato relish.

Yield: 8 servings.

Carbohydrate, 12.9 grams; Protein, 5.2 grams; Fat, 5.7 grams.
Calories, 119 per serving.

Bean Patties

¼ cup rolled oats, quick-cooking
¼ cup milk (evaporated)
1½ cups beans, mashed (without liquid)
½ teaspoon sage

2 tablespoons onions, minced
½ teaspoon salt
2 tablespoons oil or margarine

1. Combine milk and rolled oats.
2. Add minced onion, salt, and sage.
3. Add mashed beans and oil.
4. Mix lightly with fork.
5. Drop on lightly oiled skillet. Cover.
6. Let cook until well browned, and turn.
7. Cover and cook until browned.
8. Total cooking time is 6 to 8 minutes.
9. Serve plain or with tomato or cream sauce.

Yield: 4 servings.

Carbohydrate, 4.7 grams; Protein, 6.4 grams; Fat, 8.6 grams.
Calories, 120 per serving.

Beef-Style Pot Pie

1¼ cups Meatless "Beef" Style roll (see p. 174)
1 cup canned mushroom pieces
1 tablespoon margarine
1 cup carrots, crinkle cut, frozen
½ cup peas, frozen
2 medium cooking potatoes

1 tablespoon plus 1 teaspoon parsley, dry
2 tablespoons plus 2 teaspoons flour
1 teaspoon beef-like seasoning (see p. 174)
¾ cup chopped onion
2¼ cups tomato soup
5 cups mashed potatoes
1 teaspoon salt

1. Dice "Beef" Style in ½-inch cubes.
2. Drain mushrooms (save juice), and braise in margarine.
3. Cook potatoes and carrots until tender.
4. Add "Beef" Style, mushrooms, and parsley.
5. Add flour, milk, mushroom juice, and stir until smooth.
6. Add beef-like seasoning, salt, peas, and tomato soup.
7. Sauté onions, and add to mixture.
8. Pour into baking dish, and top with mashed potatoes.
9. Sprinkle with paprika, and brown lightly in hot oven.

Yield: 10 servings.

Carbohydrate, 12.9 grams; Protein, 7.4 grams; Fat, 6.4 grams.
Calories, 140 per serving.

Braised Skallops

30 Vegetable Skallops (see p. 174)
1 tablespoon brewers' yeast

2 teaspoons paprika
2 tablespoons oil

1. In hot frying pan, add oil and Skallops.
2. Sprinkle brewers' yeast and paprika on Skallops. Mix well.
3. Fry until light and crispy. Serve with gravy of your choice.

Yield: 10 servings, 3 per serving.

Carbohydrate, 3.8 grams; Protein, 11.9 grams; Fat, 4.2 grams. Calories, 99 per serving.

Cottage Cheese and Nut Loaf

1 cup cottage cheese
1 cup walnuts, chopped
1 cup bread crumbs
1 cup White Sauce (see p. 175)

2 tablespoons onion, chopped, or ¼ teaspoon onion powder
1 tablespoon margarine
2 tablespoons cottage cheese

1. Braise the onion in oil and a little water until tender.
2. Mix the other ingredients, and moisten with water in which the onion has been cooked (unless onion powder is used).
3. Pour mixture into oiled, shallow baking dish.
4. Bake in 350° oven for 45 minutes.
5. Serve with white sauce to which 2 tablespoons of cottage cheese have been added.

Yield: 6 servings.

Carbohydrate, 14.0 grams; Protein, 11.6 grams; Fat, 14.0 grams. Calories, 228 per serving.

Breaded Skallops with Tartar Sauce

2 pounds, 12 ounces
Vegetable Skallops (see
p. 174) (approximately 5½
cups)
2 eggs
⅓ cup plus 1½ teaspoons
low-fat milk

1 cup flour
Dash garlic powder
Dash seasoned salt
¾ teaspoon salt
1 teaspoon brewers' yeast
1 cup bread crumbs

1. Drain Skallops thoroughly.
2. Beat eggs, add milk, and mix.
3. Combine flour and seasonings.
4. Roll Skallops in flour mixture, then dip in egg with milk.
5. Roll in bread crumbs.
6. Deep fry to a golden brown.
7. Serve with Tartar Sauce (see p. 150).

Yield: 10 servings.

Carbohydrate, 21.2 grams; Protein, 14.7 grams; Fat, 3.6 grams.
Calories, 176 per serving.

Breaded Tastee Cuts with Brown Gravy

10 Tastee Cuts (see p. 174)
2 cups bread crumbs

1. Drain Tastee Cuts.
2. Dip in batter.
3. Roll in bread crumbs.
4. Fry on grill or frying pan.
5. Serve with Brown Gravy (see p. 175).

Batter

2 cups warm milk
1 tablespoon Vegex or
Savorex (see p. 174)

½ cup flour
3 eggs
2 teaspoons salt

1. Dissolve Vegex in warm milk, add flour, stir until smooth.
2. Add eggs, salt, and mix until smooth.

Yield: 10 servings.

Carbohydrate, 27.3 grams; Protein, 15.5 grams; Fat, 2.0 grams.
Calories, 189 per serving.

Bulgur-Chick Patties

½ cup bulgur wheat
1 cup boiling water
½ cup sautéed onions
2 tablespoons oil

1 teaspoon chicken-like seasoning
  (see p. 174)
⅛ teaspoon garlic powder
1 cup soaked garbanzos
½ cup cold water

1. Stir bulgur wheat into boiling water in a heavy saucepan.
2. Stir until evenly moistened.
3. Place on low heat.
4. Add onions, oil, and seasonings.
5. Stir with fork to mix; cook until soft.
6. Blend soaked garbanzos with cold water until fine.
7. Add to bulgur wheat, mixing well.
8. Drop from tablespoon or scoop on lightly oiled skillet.
9. Cover, bake at 350°F for 10 minutes.
10. Turn, cover, reduce heat to 325°F, and cook 15 minutes longer.
11. Serve with chopped parsley and Tahini Sauce.

Yield: 6 ½-cup servings.

Carbohydrate, 20.0 grams; Protein, 4.9 grams; Fat, 5.1 grams.
Calories, 144 per serving.

Tahini Sauce

1 cup sesame seeds
2 tablespoons oil
½ cup water

1 teaspoon salt
¼ cup lemon juice

1. Blend seeds, oil, and water until seeds are fine.
2. Add salt, lemon juice, and more water if necessary. If paste is desired, use less water.

Carbohydrate, 5.2 grams; Protein, 4.6 grams; Fat, 17.9 grams.
Calories, 200 per serving.

Carrot Loaf

3 cups grated raw carrots
2 cups cooked brown rice
1 cup raw peanuts or cashews
1 cup peanut butter

2 cups soy milk
1 tablespoon sage
1 egg, lightly beaten

1. Preheat the oven to 325°F.
2. Mix carrots, rice, and peanuts together.
3. Blend the peanut butter and soy milk.
4. Add sage and egg.
5. Pour milk mixture over carrot mixture, and mix well.
6. Turn into an oiled casserole, and bake 45 minutes or until set.

Yield: 6 servings.

Carbohydrate, 15.6 grams; Protein, 6.3 grams; Fat, 7.3 grams.
Calories, 152 per serving.

Canton Noodles with Soy Sauce

⅔ cup green onions, chopped in 1-inch lengths
3 tablespoons margarine
3 eggs, beaten
5 ounces noodles, wide (2½ cups)
¾ cup water
1 teaspoon salt
¾ cup bean sprouts
⅔ cup Vegetable Skallops (see p. 174)
¾ cup celery, sliced diagonally
¾ cup onion, sliced thin
1½ teaspoons torumel yeast
½ teaspoon salt
1 tablespoon parsley, dehydrated
2 teaspoons chicken-like seasoning (see p. 174)
¼ cup mushrooms, sliced
1 tablespoon soy sauce
¾ cup carrots

1. Grease bottom of small pan with margarine. Pour eggs into pan, and bake at 350°F for 5 minutes.
2. Cut eggs into strips 1½ inches long by ¼ inch wide.
3. Cook noodles in boiling salted water for 15 minutes. Drain and rinse in cold water.
4. Cut Skallops bite-size, and fry in an oiled pan with torumel yeast until brown.
5. Sauté onions, celery, carrots, mushrooms.
6. Add cooked noodles, seasonings, bean sprouts, green onions, and parsley. Garnish with egg strips.

Yield: 10 servings.

Carbohydrate, 13.4 grams; Protein, 5.8 grams; Fat, 6.0 grams.
Calories, 130 per serving.

Cashew Nut Casserole

¾ cup celery, diced
1 cup onions, diced
2 cups cashew pieces
15 ounces Vegetable Skallops (see p. 174), diced (approximately 1¾ cups)
2 cups cream of mushroom soup
3 tablespoons low-fat milk
2 cups chow mein noodles
1¼ teaspoons chicken-like seasoning (see p. 174)

1. Combine all ingredients.
2. Pour into an oiled pan, and bake at 300°F for 30 minutes.

Yield: 10 servings.

Carbohydrate, 16.7 grams; Protein, 9.9 grams; Fat, 17.1 grams.
Calories, 250 per serving.

Cashew Nut Loaf

½ pound cashews
¾ cup onions
¾ cup milk
¾ teaspoon paprika
1½ cups Vege-Burger (see p. 174)
1½ cups plus 1 tablespoon bread crumbs
4 eggs

1 teaspoon Vegex, melted (see p. 174)
3 tablespoons margarine, melted
1 tablespoon parsley
1 teaspoon celery salt
1½ teaspoons Bakon Yeast (see p. 174)
1 teaspoon sage
1 teaspoon salt
1½ tablespoons vegetable oil

1. Put nuts and onions through food chopper, coarse blade.
2. Combine all ingredients, and mix well.
3. Place mixture in oiled pan.
4. Bake 45 to 60 minutes at 350°F.
5. Serve with mushroom sauce (1 part mushroom soup to 2 parts White Sauce, see p. 175).

Yield: 10 servings.

Carbohydrate, 26.4 grams; Protein, 12.2 grams; Fat, 18.0 grams. Calories, 317 per serving.

Chili Relleno

9 egg whites
2 eggs, beaten
¼ teaspoon salt

8 ounces jack cheese, cut in slices 3½ × ½ inches
10 green, canned chilies

1. Beat egg whites until stiff.
2. Fold in beaten eggs.
3. Add seasonings, and set aside.
4. Stuff chilies with jack cheese slices.
5. Place stuffed chilies on bun pan and pour egg mixture on top.
6. Bake in oven at 350°F until golden brown.
7. Serve with tomato sauce.

Tomato Sauce

1 tablespoon oil
¼ cup onions, chopped
¼ cup green peppers, chopped
2 cups tomato soup

2 tablespoons water
¼ teaspoon salt
¼ teaspoon garlic powder

1. Sauté onions and green pepper in oil.
2. Add tomato soup, water, and seasonings. Simmer.

Yield: 10 servings.

Carbohydrate, 1.6 grams; Protein, 12.4 grams; Fat, 7.8 grams. Calories, 126 per serving.

Cheese Blintzes with Strawberry Sauce

Batter

7 eggs
½ cup milk
2 tablespoons oil

1 tablespoon flour
1 teaspoon salt

1. Beat eggs.
2. Beat milk, flour, salt, and oil until smooth.
3. Add eggs to milk mixture.
4. Into 6-inch frying pan, pour 1 teaspoon oil, and heat on top of stove.
5. Put 3 tablespoons egg batter in pan.
6. After batter is light brown, flip it over and place it immediately on paper to cool.

Filling

½ cup hoop cheese (dry, non-fat cottage cheese)
1½ cups cream cheese

2 tablespoons flour
1 teaspoon salt

1. Combine cheeses.
2. Add flour and salt.
3. Mix until smooth.
4. Put 2 tablespoons of cheese mixture on brown side of pancake.
5. Roll like a jelly roll.
6. Fry in well-greased, medium-hot frying pan. Fry on both sides.
7. Serve with hot strawberry sauce.

Yield: 10 servings.

Strawberry Sauce

1 cup strawberry syrup
2 cups frozen strawberries

¼ cup cornstarch

1. Thaw strawberries, drain, and save juice.
2. Bring the juice and syrup to a boil.
3. Dissolve cornstarch in water, and thicken the juice.
4. Add strawberries and heat.

Blintzes only:
Carbohydrate, 3.3 grams; Protein, 9.0 grams; Fat, 13.8 grams.
Calories, 175 per serving.

Chinese Spinach and Noodles

1 8-ounce package spinach (or beet leaves)
6 Dinner Cuts, cut into strips (see p. 174)
2 cups Chinese white flat noodles (or substitute), cooked
1 clove garlic, crushed
2 teaspoons soy sauce
1 8-ounce can sliced mushrooms
1 cup sliced onion
1 teaspoon salt
2 tablespoons flour

1. Sauté onion in oil for a few minutes, then add mushrooms, garlic, and strips of Dinner Cuts which have been previously dipped in flour.
2. Cut spinach or beet leaves finely, and cook in a little water for 5 minutes.
3. Put noodles in hot, salted water, and cook for 3 minutes.
4. When ingredients in the fry pan are nicely browned and cooked, add the spinach or beet leaves, soy sauce, salt, and noodles.
5. Heat and serve immediately.

Yield: 8 servings.

Carbohydrate, 11.0 grams; Protein, 7.8 grams; Fat, 4.5 grams. Calories, 116 per serving.

Chop Suey with Rice

1 can Tastee Cuts (see p. 174)
1 tablespoon brewers' yeast
2 cups celery, chopped
2 cups onions
1 cup green onions
1½ cups mushrooms, sliced
1 cup bamboo shoots, sliced
1 cup water chestnuts
2 cups bean sprouts
½ pound margarine
4 tablespoons soy sauce
3 tablespoons corn starch

1. Drain Tastee Cuts, and save juice.
2. Cut Tastee Cuts 1 inch × ¼ inch.
3. Braise cuts with brewers' yeast in a little oil.
4. Cook celery, onions, green onions, and margarine with liquid from the Tastee Cuts, bamboo shoots, and water chestnuts.
5. Add soy sauce.
6. Dissolve corn starch in a little water and liquid from the Tastee Cuts mixture to thicken.
7. Add bean sprouts and heat.
8. Serve on cooked hot brown or white rice.
9. Substitute Chinese noodles in place of rice for Chow Mein.

Yield: 10 servings.

Carbohydrate, 29.9 grams; Protein, 9.5 grams; Fat, 6.4 grams. Calories, 216 per serving.

Corn Fritters

2 cups cream-style corn
2 cups flour
1 tablespoon sugar
1 tablespoon baking powder
5 eggs
1 teaspoon salt
1 quart oil for frying

1. Mix all ingredients. Form into balls using 3 level tablespoons of mixture for each ball.
2. Deep fry at 350°F.
3. Put in 300°F oven for 20 minutes.
4. Serve with syrup.

Yield: 10 servings.

Carbohydrate, 26.8 grams; Protein, 5.4 grams; Fat, 3.0 grams.
Calories, 156 per serving.

Chinese-Style Sautéed Tofu

1½ pounds tofu, steamed
2 tablespoons oil
½ teaspoon salt
1 small onion, thinly sliced
6 mushrooms
1 small carrot, cut into thin strips
2 green peppers, cut into thin strips
1½ stalks celery, cut into diagonal, thin slices
½ cup bamboo shoots
1½ tablespoons soy sauce
1 teaspoon grated ginger root
1 tablespoon sugar
1 tablespoon water
2 teaspoons cornstarch, dissolved in 6 tablespoons water

1. Cut tofu crosswise into pieces.
2. Heat skillet, coat with the oil, and sprinkle on the salt.
3. Add onion, then the mushrooms; stir fry over high heat for about 30 seconds.
4. Reduce heat to medium low; add carrot, green pepper, celery, bamboo shoots, and tofu in that order, sautéing each for about 1 minute.
5. Reduce heat to low; add soy sauce, ginger root, sugar, and water.
6. Simmer for 3 to 4 minutes. Stir in dissolved cornstarch, and simmer for 30 seconds more.

Yield: 4 servings.

Carbohydrate, 18.6 grams; Protein, 16.0 grams; Fat, 6.0 grams.
Calories, 190 per serving.

Chili with Beans

2¼ cups pinto beans
7 cups boiling water
3½ cups cooked tomatoes
½ cup tomato paste
1 cup sautéed onions
2 tablespoons oil
1 tablespoon sugar

½ tablespoon salt
¼ teaspoon oregano
1 cup Vege-Burger (see p. 174)
¼ teaspoon cumin
½ teaspoon sweet basil
¼ teaspoon garlic powder

1. Cook beans in water until tender..
2. When tender, add salt, sugar, onions, tomatoes, Vege-Burger, oil, and tomato paste.
3. Simmer until liquid is evaporated to a thick consistency.
4. Add herbs and garlic powder.
5. Simmer 20 minutes more.
6. Serve with crackers or zwieback.

Yield: 6 1-cup servings.

Carbohydrate, 30.4 grams; Protein, 13.8 grams; Fat, 18.2 grams.
Calories, 341 per serving.

Cheese and Nut Loaf

2 cups cottage cheese
1 cup grated cheese
1 cup nuts, roasted and chopped
¼ cup onions, chopped and braised

¼ cup celery, finely diced
6 eggs
¾ cup bread crumbs
1 tablespoon soy sauce
Dash garlic powder

1. Mix all ingredients.
2. Pour into oiled pan.
3. Put in double pan with water in it.
4. Bake in 325°F oven for 1½ hours.
5. Slice in 10 pieces, and serve with Brown Gravy (see p. 175).

Yield: 10 servings.

Carbohydrate, 9.6 grams; Protein, 14.9 grams; Fat, 16.5 grams.
Calories, 244 per serving.

Cottage Cheese Patties

1 cup cottage cheese	6 eggs
1 cup ground whole-wheat crackers or bread crumbs	½ teaspoon sage
	¼ teaspoon salt
1 cup walnuts, chopped	1 onion, finely chopped

1. Mix together all ingredients in order given.
2. Shape into patties.
3. Fry in skillet with oil or Pam until light brown.
4. May be eaten like this or may cover with one can of cream of mushroom soup diluted with ¾ can of water, and baked at 325°F for 20 to 30 minutes.

Yield: 8 servings.

Carbohydrate, 7.5 grams; Protein, 13.2 grams; Fat, 13.2 grams.
Calories, 202 per serving.

Creamed Chipped Beef-Style on Rusk

½ pound Corned "Beef"-Style roll (see p. 174)	⅛ teaspoon ground celery seed
2½ teaspoons oil	⅝ teaspoon onion powder
3¼ cups low-fat milk	⅝ teaspoon torumel yeast
3½ tablespoons margarine	⅝ teaspoon salt
¼ cup flour	10 slices Holland rusk

1. Dice Corned "Beef"-Style coarsely.
2. Place on oiled sheet pan, separating the pieces as much as possible.
3. Sprinkle oil on top.
4. Brown in oven at 350°F for approximately 15 minutes.
5. Heat milk.
6. Melt margarine, add flour and seasonings, stir until smooth.
7. Add hot milk gradually, stirring constantly.
8. Cook and stir as necessary until smooth and thickened.
9. Pour White Sauce (see p. 175) over Corned "Beef"-Style, gently folding in the sauces.
10. Serve on rusk or toast.

Yield: 10 servings.

Carbohydrate, 16.2 grams; Protein, 8.4 grams; Fat, 10.3 grams.
Calories, 192 per serving.

Creamed Chow Mein and Rice

5 Tastee Cuts (see p. 174)
1 teaspoon brewers' yeast
1 cup drained mushrooms
½ cup oil
2 tablespoons flour
4 cups hot milk
½ cup onions, sliced and braised
½ cup green onions, sliced and braised
½ cup celery, sliced and braised
1 cup whole roasted cashews
2 tablespoons soy sauce
1 teaspoon salt
6 cups cooked rice

1. Cut Tastee Cuts in half and cut in ¼-inch strips.
2. Braise the Tastee Cuts in a little oil and brewers' yeast.
3. Make mushroom cream sauce with mushrooms, oil, flour, and hot milk.
4. Mix all ingredients.
5. Heat and serve over hot rice.

Yield: 10 servings.

Carbohydrate, 25.7 grams; Protein, 8.5 grams; Fat, 20.9 grams.
Calories, 323 per serving.

Egg a la King on Toast

10 hard-cooked eggs, diced
4 tablespoons margarine
½ cup mushrooms
2 tablespoons flour
3 cups milk
1 teaspoon chicken-flavor seasoning (see p. 174)
½ teaspoon salt
½ cup peas
½ cup onions, diced and braised
1 tablespoon pimento, diced
10 pieces toast

1. Braise mushrooms in margarine.
2. Add flour; stir well.
3. Add milk; stir until smooth.
4. Add remaining ingredients except toast, and heat well.
5. Serve on toast.

Yield: 10 servings.

Carbohydrate, 23.0 grams; Protein, 16.0 grams; Fat, 14.0 grams.
Calories, 282 per serving.

Egg Croquettes with Brown Gravy

8 hard-cooked eggs
1 tablespoon onions,
 chopped and braised
1 tablespoon bell peppers,
 chopped and braised
1 teaspoon pimento, diced
½ cup milk

2 eggs, raw
1 cup White Sauce, thick (see p. 175)
1 teaspoon brewers' yeast
1½ cups cornflake crumbs
2 quarts oil—enough for deep-fat
 frying

1. Chop cooked eggs, coarsely.
2. Reserve ½ cup of the cornflake crumbs.
3. Combine all ingredients.
4. Measure 3 tablespoons of mixture, make cone-shaped croquettes.
5. Dip in milk and cornflake crumbs.
6. Chill overnight.
7. Roll in cornflake crumbs again.
8. Deep fry in oil.
9. May serve with Brown Gravy (see p. 175).

Yield: 10 servings.

Carbohydrate, 12.4 grams; Protein, 12.0 grams; Fat, 15.8 grams.
Calories, 244 per serving.

Egg Foo Yung—Low Cholesterol

¼ cup plus 1½ tablespoons
 celery, sliced
¼ cup plus 2½ tablespoons
 bean sprouts, fresh
¼ cup plus 1½ tablespoons
 green onions, freshly
 chopped
½ cup plus 1½ tablespoons
 water chestnuts, sliced

1 cup eggs, low cholesterol
¾ cup plus 1½ tablespoons mushroom
 pieces
½ teaspoon salt
⅜ teaspoon soy sauce
1½ teaspoons oil

1. Combine all ingredients, except oil, in mixing bowl. Mix well.
2. Pour oil in hot frying pan.
3. Fry ¼ cup portions until brown.

Yield: 8 (3.1 ounce) servings.

Carbohydrate, 4.7 grams; Protein, 6.5 grams; Fat, 8.7 grams.
Calories, 123 per serving.

Egg Foo Yung

12 eggs
1 cup celery, chopped
1 cup onions, chopped
¾ cup green onions, chopped

½ pound bean sprouts
⅓ cup soy sauce
1 cup mushrooms

1. Beat eggs.
2. Add ingredients.
3. Heat frying pan, add oil.
4. Shape mixture into 10 patties, place in oiled pan, and bake 12–15 minutes in 350°F oven (patties may be fried on low heat).

Yield: 10 servings.

Carbohydrate, 4.7 grams; Protein, 6.5 grams; Fat, 8.7 grams.
Calories, 123 per serving.

Egg, Mushroom, and Pea Casserole

3 tablespoons margarine
¼ cup flour
¼ teaspoon salt
1½ cups milk
4 cups peas
6 eggs, hard-boiled, quartered

4 cups celery, diced
1 small can mushrooms
¼ cup green peppers, diced
½ cup pimento, diced
1 can Chinese noodles (2½ ounce can)

1. Make white sauce of first four ingredients.
2. Add in next six ingredients.
3. Simmer 30 minutes.
4. Arrange in casserole, and garnish with noodles.

Yield: 10 servings.

Carbohydrate, 23.6 grams; Protein, 10.4 grams; Fat, 10.4 grams.
Calories, 225 per serving.

Eggplant Casserole

1½ pounds eggplant, diced
2 tablespoons margarine
½ cup onions, diced
2 tomatoes, sliced

⅔ cup cream of tomato soup
1½ teaspoons salt
1 cup Cheddar cheese, shredded
¾ cup sour cream

1. Steam eggplant until tender. Drain.
2. Sauté onions in margarine until soft.
3. Combine eggplant, onion, tomatoes, tomato soup, and salt.
4. Fold in sour cream.
5. Top with Cheddar cheese.
6. Bake until bubbly and cheese is melted.

Yield: 10 servings.

Carbohydrate, 7.8 grams; Protein, 4.8 grams; Fat, 9.9 grams.
Calories, 136 per serving.

Enchiladas

12 tortillas
1 pound shredded American
  cheese
¼ cup minced olives

½ cup onions, chopped and braised
4 cups tomato sauce
2 ounces melted margarine

1. Mix 12 ounces cheese, olives, onions, and melted margarine to a light creamy texture.
2. Spoon cheese mixture on tortilla and roll tortilla around the mixture.
3. Place enchilada in oiled pan.
4. Pour tomato sauce over enchiladas.
5. Sprinkle sauce with 4 ounces of grated cheese.
6. Bake in 350°F oven until light brown.

Yield: 12 servings.

Carbohydrate, 6.5 grams; Protein, 10.8 grams; Fat, 14.8 grams.
Calories, 201 per serving.

Fried Tofu Patties with Eggs and Vegetables

1½ pounds tofu, drained
Thin tips and leaves of one
  stalk of celery, minced
1 small onion, minced
2 tablespoons green onions,
  chopped
¼ cup carrots, coarsely
  shredded

4 eggs, lightly beaten
1 teaspoon salt
2 tablespoons soy sauce
½ cup bread crumbs
4 tablespoons oil

1. In a large bowl combine the nine ingredients. Mix well.
2. Form into patties.
3. Fry in hot oil until nicely browned.
4. Top with a mixture of ¼ cup catsup and 2 tablespoons soy sauce.

Yield: 15 to 20 patties.

15 patties
Carbohydrate, 3.0 grams; Protein, 5.7 grams; Fat, 7.0 grams. Calories, 95 per serving.

20 patties
Carbohydrate, 2.3 grams; Protein, 4.3 grams; Fat, 5.4 grams. Calories, 71 per serving.

Garbanzo Burgers

2 cups soaked garbanzos
¾ cup water
2 tablespoons soy sauce
1 small onion, chopped fine,
  or ½ teaspoon onion
  powder

1½ cups soaked soybeans
1 teaspoon beef-like seasoning (see
  p. 174)
Sprinkle of garlic powder
Salt if necessary
½ cup water

1. Combine soaked garbanzos, ¾ cup water, onion, and other seasonings.
2. Blend until medium fine.
3. Pour into bowl.
4. Blend soybeans with ½ cup water until medium fine.
5. Add to garbanzo mixture.
6. Dip one-half cup of mixture, and shape for pattie.
7. Fry in oiled pan.
8. Cover, let cook 10 minutes or until nicely browned.
9. Turn, cover, let cook for 10 minutes.
10. Reduce heat, let cook for an additional 10 minutes.

Note: Chicken-like seasoning may be used instead of beef-like seasoning. May be baked as a loaf or casserole.

Yield: 8 servings.

Carbohydrate, 15.7 grams; Protein, 10.4 grams; Fat, 5.4 grams. Calories, 152 per serving.

Garbanzo-Pimento Cheese

1 cup garbanzos, soaked
⅓ cup brazil nuts
¼ cup brewers' yeast
4-ounce jar pimentos
½ teaspoon onion powder

⅛ teaspoon garlic powder
¼ cup lemon juice
1½ cups water
1 teaspoon salt

1. Soak garbanzos 24 hours in 3 cups water.
2. Drain off soaking water.
3. Scrape off brown husk from brazil nuts, and cut into medium-size pieces.
4. Combine all the ingredients in blender.
5. Blend until very fine.
6. Mix in bowl, then place in kettle.
7. Cook covered 25 to 30 minutes or longer. Stir occasionally.
8. Mold in two small bread pans that have been rinsed with cold water.
9. Chill, unmold, slice, and serve.

Note: Garbanzo-Herb Cheese: Substitute fresh chives and sage or other herbs for pimentos.

Yield: 12 servings.

Carbohydrate, 13.7 grams; Protein, 6.1 grams; Fat, 6.3 grams.
Calories, 136 per serving.

Garbanzo Stew and Dumplings

6 cups garbanzos, canned
6 scrambled eggs, chopped
1 cup onions, chopped and
braised

1 tablespoon chicken-like seasoning
(see p. 174)
1 teaspoon salt, if garbanzos aren't salty
1 tablespoon cornstarch

1. Combine all ingredients except cornstarch. Bring to a boil.
2. Dissolve cornstarch in water, use to thicken garbanzo mixture.

Dumplings

4 cups flour
¼ cup vegetable shortening
1 tablespoon baking powder
1 teaspoon sugar
¾ teaspoon salt

4 eggs
2 cups milk
½ cup parsley
1½ cups chicken-like broth (see
p. 174)
Pinch yellow coloring

1. Mix all ingredients except broth.
2. Bring broth to boil.
3. Measure ¼ cup of dumpling dough and drop it in boiling broth; repeat until dough is gone.
4. Place dumplings on garbanzo stew, and serve hot.

Yield: 10 servings.

Carbohydrate, 57.0 grams; Protein, 19.0 grams; Fat, 21.0 grams.
Calories, 490 per serving.

Granola and Sweet-Corn Roast

1 cup granola	½ cup walnuts, finely chopped
1 cup milk	1 tablespoon soy flour
2 eggs	½ teaspoon oregano
8 ounces sweet-corn, cream style	1 teaspoon parsley
1 grated onion	1 teaspoon salt

1. Place granola and salt in a bowl, and cover with boiling water.
2. Stir and let swell for 10 minutes.
3. Add corn, beaten eggs, and other ingredients.
4. Pour mixture into oiled baking dish, and bake in a moderate oven for 45 minutes to 1 hour.
5. Serve hot or cold.
6. Cuts nicely if left in the refrigerator until cold.

Yield: 8 servings.

Carbohydrate, 12.6 grams; Protein, 5.3 grams; Fat, 8.0 grams. Calories, 332 per serving.

Grape-Nuts Roast

1 cup Grape-Nuts cereal	1 cup chopped walnuts
2 eggs, beaten	½ chopped onion, medium size
1½ cups skim milk	1 cup chopped celery
½ teaspoon salt	2 tablespoons melted margarine
1 can mushroom soup, condensed	

1. Combine all ingredients.
2. Let stand 20 minutes.
3. Pour into greased loaf pan. Bake at 350°F for 1 hour.

Yield: 6 servings.

Carbohydrate, 22.7 grams; Protein, 9.8 grams; Fat, 22.4 grams. Calories, 332 per serving.

Grain-Nut Burger

1 cup raw oats
½ to 1 cup water-cooked oats
¾ cup bread crumbs
1 sautéed onion
3 eggs
1 cup cooked brown rice
¼ cup oil
1 teaspoon brewers' yeast

1 teaspoon sage
2 teaspoons Savorex (see p. 174)
1 tablespoon beef-like seasoning (see p. 174)
½ teaspoon salt
3 ounces chopped walnuts
¼ cup hot water
1 teaspoon soy sauce

1. Combine all ingredients.
2. Shape into patties.
3. Fry on grill.

Yield: 15 servings.

Carbohydrate, 13.3 grams; Protein, 4.8 grams; Fat, 8.8 grams. Calories, 148 per serving.

Imperial Roast with Brown Gravy

2½ cups brown rice, cooked
1 cup walnuts, chopped
1½ cups Vege-Burger (see p. 174)
½ cup onions, chopped and braised
1 cup bread crumbs

¾ cup half-and-half cream
5 eggs
1 teaspoon Vegex (see p. 174)
1 tablespoon vegetable shortening
2 cups Brown Gravy (see p. 175)

1. Mix all ingredients.
2. Pour mixture in a pan lined with oiled paper.
3. Brush with melted margarine.
4. Put in double pan with water in bottom pan.
5. Bake in 300°F oven for 1¼ hours.
6. Serve with Brown Gravy.

Yield: 10 servings.

Carbohydrate, 20.9 grams; Protein, 13.7 grams; Fat, 13.1 grams. Calories, 257 per serving.

Leafy Chinese Tofu

1 pound tofu, cut into 1-inch
  cubes
1 tablespoon oil
½ pound spinach or any leafy
  green vegetable, torn into
  bite-size pieces

½ cup sesame seeds
3 tablespoons soy sauce
1 cup raw brown rice, cooked, cold

1. Put 1 tablespoon of oil in large frying pan.
2. Sauté tofu cubes about 5 minutes.
3. Push the cubes to the center of the pan, and spread the torn spinach all around the edge.
4. Sprinkle the tofu with sesame seeds and half the soy sauce.
5. Cover the pan to steam the spinach until it is just wilted. Be careful not to overcook it.
6. Remove from heat, and drain excess liquid.
7. Sprinkle remaining soy sauce over the spinach, and serve with rice.

Yield: 8 servings.

Carbohydrate, 14.1 grams; Protein, 8.3 grams; Fat, 9.6 grams.
Calories, 175 per serving.

Lentil-Carrot Loaf

2 cups cooked lentils
1 cup powdered skim milk in
  ⅔ cup water
2 cups carrots, grated
1 cup celery, chopped
½ cup onion, chopped

¼ cup oil
1 egg
½ teaspoon sage
½ teaspoon salt
¼ cup cooked carrot slices

1. Mash lentils.
2. Mix all remaining ingredients except carrot slices.
3. Bake in a greased 9 × 9 pan at 350°F for 45 minutes.
4. Cut into squares; arrange on platter.
5. Garnish with cooked carrot slices.

Yield: 9 servings.

Carbohydrate, 19.3 grams; Protein, 9.4 grams; Fat, 6.8 grams.
Calories, 173 per serving

Lentil and Rice Loaf

2 cups steamed rice
1 cup lentils
1 tablespoon onion, chopped
2 tablespoons margarine or oil

1 tablespoon browned flour
⅓ cup tomato juice
Salt and sage to taste

1. Sauté onions in a small pan until golden in color.
2. Add flour and tomato juice; stir until smooth.
3. Mix together with rice, lentils, and seasonings.
4. Place in oiled baking dish, and bake for 30–35 minutes at 375°F.
5. Additional tomato juice and grated cheese may be added as topping before baking.

Yield: 6 ½-cup servings.

Carbohydrate, 19.5 grams; Protein, 3.9 grams; Fat, 5.0 grams.
Calories, 139 per serving.

Lentil-Walnut Patties

3 cups lentils, cooked
2 cups walnuts, roasted
½ cup onions, chopped and braised

5 eggs
1 cup bread crumbs
½ cup tomato sauce
1 teaspoon salt

1. Grind the lentils coarsely.
2. Chop walnuts coarsely.
3. Mix all ingredients.
4. Grease baking sheet.
5. Make patties on baking sheet, measuring ¼ cup.
6. Bake in 325°F oven for 20 minutes.
7. Serve with Brown Gravy or Mushroom Gravy (see p. 175).

Yield: 10 servings.

Carbohydrate, 21.0 grams; Protein, 12.7 grams; Fat, 19.5 grams.
Calories 314 per serving.

Maritime Patties with Tartar Sauce

1 pound White Chix (see p. 174)
7 ounce-can Tartex (see p. 174)
¼ cup mayonnaise
3 eggs, raw
½ cup onions, chopped and braised
¼ cup celery, chopped
2 tablespoons parsley, chopped
2 tablespoons pimento, chopped
1 tablespoon chicken-like seasoning (see p. 174)
1½ cups cornflake crumbs

1. Coarsely grind the White Chix.
2. Combine all ingredients with 1 cup cornflake crumbs.
3. Make patties, and roll in ½ cup cornflake crumbs.
4. Deep fry.
5. Serve with Tartar Sauce (see p. 150).

Yield: 10 servings.

Carbohydrate, 16.0 grams; Protein, 12.7 grams; Fat, 19.9 grams.
Calories, 293 per serving.

Tartar Sauce: per tablespoon.

Carbohydrate, 1.0 gram; Protein, .4 gram; Fat, 4.0 grams.
Calories, 41 per tablespoon.

Maritime Roast

1 pound FriChik, ground (see p. 174)
1 7-ounce can Tartex (see p. 174)
1 tablespoon onion, ground
½ cup salad dressing
½ teaspoon paprika
3 sticks celery, ground
2 eggs, beaten
4 raw potatoes, ground

1. Combine all ingredients. If mixture is a little thin, add a few bread crumbs.
2. Place in buttered casserole.
3. Bake at 350°F for 45 minutes to 1 hour.

Yield: 10 servings.

Carbohydrate, 17.0 grams; Protein, 19.0 grams; Fat, 15.0 grams.
Calories, 280 per serving.

Mediterranean Stuffed Swiss Chard Leaves

½ pound fresh Swiss chard or grape leaves
1 pound ricotta cheese
½ cup raisins
½ cup sunflower seeds
¼ cup cashew nuts, chopped
½ cup fresh mushrooms, chopped
½ teaspoon nutmeg
¼ teaspoon tarragon
1 tablespoon sunflower seed oil
1 onion, finely chopped
Salt to taste

1. Select the best chard leaves, preferably all the same size. Wash and remove white stems.
2. Steam the leaves until they are soft but retain their green color.
3. Set aside to cool.
4. Sauté onion and mushrooms for 5 minutes in 1 tablespoon of oil.
5. Combine mushrooms and onion with ricotta cheese along with the rest of ingredients, and blend.
6. Stuff leaves uniformly by placing 2–3 tablespoons of filling in the center of each leaf, the vein side up. Fold sides over first, then the top and bottom of leaves to form a flat envelope shape.
7. Place stuffed leaves, smooth side up, side by side, in an oiled baking pan (use 3 tablespoons of oil on bottom of pan). Do not place them on top of each other.
8. Brush top of each leaf with oil.
9. Bake, covered, so leaves do not burn, in preheated oven at 350°F for 30 minutes.
10. Remove cover and bake uncovered for 15 minutes more.
11. Serve hot.

Yield: 8 servings.

Carbohydrate, 14.5 grams; Protein, 12.1 grams; Fat, 10.8 grams.
Calories, 203 per serving.

Mushroom Loaf with Brown Gravy

1 cup mushrooms, canned
1 cup potatoes, shredded
½ cup onions, chopped and braised
½ cup half-and-half cream
1 can Vege-Burger (see p. 174)
6 eggs
1 tablespoon chicken-like seasoning (see p. 174)
1 teaspoon salt
½ cup bread crumbs
2 cups Brown Gravy (see p. 175)

1. Grind mushrooms coarsely.
2. Mix all ingredients.
3. Pour into oiled pan.
4. Bake at 350°F for 1 hour.
5. Serve with Brown Gravy.

Yield: 10 servings.

Carbohydrate, 8.1 grams; Protein, 11.8 grams; Fat, 4.8 grams.
Calories, 124 per serving.

Noodle Supreme

4 cups noodles, cooked
½ cup mushrooms, raw
1 cup cream-of-mushroom soup, condensed
1 cup cream-of-tomato soup, condensed
½ cup sour cream
½ cup half-and-half cream
½ cup onions, chopped and braised
1 cup peas, frozen, cooked

1. Mix all ingredients.
2. Pour in casserole.
3. Bake in 350°F oven for 45 minutes.

Yield: 10 servings.

Carbohydrate, 23.9 grams; Protein, 5.3 grams; Fat, 7.2 grams. Calories, 179 per serving.

Nut-Fish Patties

1 19-ounce can Nuteena (see p. 174)
2 tablespoons peanut butter
1½ cups mashed potato
1 egg, beaten
⅔ cup soft bread crumbs
1 teaspoon parsley, freshly chopped
1 tablespoon onion, chopped
½ teaspoon salt
½ cup dried bread crumbs.

1. Mash Nuteena with fork.
2. Mix all ingredients (except dried bread crumbs) thoroughly.
3. Form mixture into small balls, and roll in dried bread crumbs.
4. Press out to ¾ inch thickness.
5. Brown both sides in small amount of oil.

Yield: 10 servings.

Carbohydrate, 11.1 grams; Protein, 9.3 grams; Fat, 12.6 grams. Calories, 194 per serving.

Nuteena a la King

7 ounces Nuteena (see p. 174)
¼ cup onions, chopped
¼ cup green onions, chopped
3 eggs, hard-cooked, diced
½ cup frozen peas
1 tablespoon parsley, chopped
3 cups White Sauce (see p. 175)
1 cup mushrooms
¼ pound margarine
8 melba toast slices

1. Braise onions, green onions, and mushrooms in margarine.
2. Add remaining ingredients, and heat.
3. Serve on Melba toast.

Yield: 8 servings.

Carbohydrate, 48.0 grams; Protein, 14.5 grams; Fat, 17.0 grams. Calories, 405 per serving.

Oatburgers

1 cup rolled oats, more
   tender if oats have been
   precooked
1 cup cottage cheese
1 cup cornflakes, crushed

2 eggs
Salt, onion salt, garlic salt, and sage to
   taste
2 tablespoons oil
1 can cream-of-mushroom soup

1. Mix above ingredients together, and form into small balls.
2. Brown lightly in oil, and put in baking dish.
3. Pour one can of cream-of-mushroom soup over balls. The cream-of-mushroom soup may be diluted with about ¼ soup-can of milk.
4. Bake in covered dish at 350°F for about 30 minutes.

Yield: 6 servings.

Carbohydrate, 14.2 grams; Protein, 9.4 grams; Fat, 11.4 grams.
Calories, 198 per serving.

Olive Patties

1 cup pitted olives, coarsely
   ground
1 cup rice, cooked
1 cup rolled oats
¼ cup onions, chopped and
   braised

6 eggs
½ teaspoon salt
Dash sweet basil

1. Mix all ingredients.
2. Let stand ½ hour.
3. Make patties.
4. Fry on grill, and put in oven for 20 minutes at 350°F.
5. Serve with Mushroom Gravy or White Sauce (see p. 175).

Yield: 10 servings.

Carbohydrate, 10.0 grams; Protein, 6.1 grams; Fat, 11.8 grams.
Calories, 170 per serving.

Oriental Noodles

4 cups egg-enriched noodles,
   cooked
1 cup fresh mushrooms
¼ cup margarine
1 cup onions, chopped and
   braised

4 eggs
1 cup peas
1 teaspoon salt

1. Braise mushrooms in margarine.
2. Beat eggs; add to mushrooms, and brown slightly.
3. Add remaining ingredients. Mix well.
4. Put mixture in pan and heat in oven at 350°F for 10 minutes.

Yield: 10 servings.

Carbohydrate, 19.8 grams; Protein, 6.9 grams; Fat, 8.3 grams.
Calories, 182 per serving.

Oriental Rice

4 cups rice, cooked, white or natural
1 cup mushrooms
4 eggs
1 cup onions, chopped and braised

½ teaspoon salt
4 tablespoons margarine
1 cup peas

1. Braise mushrooms in margarine.
2. Beat eggs; add to mushrooms, and brown slightly.
3. Add remaining ingredients. Mix well.
4. Refry mixture, and serve hot.

Yield: 10 servings.

Carbohydrate, 9.8 grams; Protein, 4.6 grams; Fat, 5.0 grams. Calories, 103 per serving.

Oriental Stew on Rice or Chinese Noodles

8 ounces steamed tofu
½ cup green onions, diced
1 cup onions, diced
1 cup celery, diced
¼ cup soy sauce

1 tablespoon brewers' yeast
2 tablespoons cornstarch
¼ pound margarine
2 tablespoons oil

1. Dice tofu into ½ inch squares.
2. Sprinkle the tofu with brewers' yeast, and fry in 2 tablespoons oil.
3. Cover vegetables with water. Add soy sauce and margarine.
4. When done, dissolve cornstarch with water, and thicken vegetables.
5. Add diced tofu, and mix lightly.
6. Serve on rice or Chinese noodles.

Yield: 8 ½-cup servings.

Carbohydrate, 8.4 grams; Protein, 3.7 grams; Fat, 12.9 grams. Calories, 165 per serving.

Peas and Barley Casserole

2 tablespoons oil
1 onion, finely chopped
½ cup yellow split peas,
  washed and drained
2½ cups broth, chicken-
  flavor (see p. 174)
¼ cup soy grits—not
  concentrated

½ cup whole barley, washed and
  drained
2 tablespoons chopped parsley
3 tablespoons dill weed
Salt to taste
¼ pound canned mushrooms, sliced

1. Heat the oil in a heavy saucepan, and sauté the onion in it until tender.
2. Add the split peas and cook 3 minutes.
3. Meanwhile, add one half cup broth to grits. Set aside.
4. Add barley to saucepan, and cook 2 minutes, stirring occasionally.
5. Add remaining broth, soaked grits, the parsley, dill, and salt.
6. Bring to a boil and simmer, covered, until liquid has been absorbed and barley is tender, about 55 minutes.
7. Add mushrooms. Cook 5 minutes longer.

Yield: 4 servings.

Carbohydrate, 45.5 grams; Protein, 10.0 grams; Fat, 7.5 grams.
Calories, 290 per serving.

Peanut-Carrot Roast

1 cup peanuts
1 cup garbanzos, soaked
1 cup water
2 cups cooked brown rice
2 cups raw carrots, shredded

1 cup sautéed onions
1 teaspoon salt, or to taste
Dash garlic powder
Few sprigs parsley

1. Place peanuts, garbanzos, and water in blender, and chop fine.
2. Add remaining ingredients. Mix well.
3. Bake in greased dish 8 × 12 inches at 350°F for 45 minutes, covered for the first 30 minutes, uncovered for the last 15 minutes.
4. Garnish with parsley, and serve hot.

Yield: 12 servings.

Carbohydrate, 16.3 grams; Protein, 6.3 grams; Fat, 9.0 grams.
Calories, 171 per serving.

Pecan Loaf

2 tablespoons oil
1 tablespoon onion, chopped
½ cup celery, chopped
1½ cups milk
1 teaspoon salt

½ cup pecans, chopped
1 cup whole-wheat bread crumbs
¼ cup parsley, chopped
2 eggs or 2 scant tablespoons soy flour

1. Heat the oil in a skillet.
2. Add the onion and celery. Steam a few minutes.
3. Add the milk and salt.
4. Remove from heat, and add the soft bread crumbs, pecans, parsley, and beaten eggs.
5. Bake in oiled loaf pan in moderate oven until set, about 1 hour.

Yield: 6 servings.

Carbohydrate, 21.0 grams; Protein, 9.5 grams; Fat, 21.0 grams.
Calories, 311 per serving.

Piquant Balls with Sour Cream Gravy

3 cups Prime, slices or roll
  (see p. 174)
½ cup Vege-Burger (see
  p. 174)
4 eggs

1 cup half-and-half cream
¼ cup onions, chopped and braised
¾ cup cornflake crumbs

1. Mix all ingredients.
2. Make mixture into balls.
3. Deep fry.

Sour Cream Gravy

4 tablespoons margarine
¾ cup milk or George
  Washington Broth
¼ cup onions, sliced and
  braised

1 teaspoon chicken-like seasoning
  (see p. 174)
1½ cups sour cream
1 tablespoon flour

1. Prepare a light gravy with margarine and hot milk or George Washington Broth.
2. Add remaining ingredients, and heat well.
3. Pour over the piquant balls, and heat in 300°F oven for 15 to 20 minutes.

Yield: 10 servings.

Carbohydrate, 16.0 grams; Protein, 15.7 grams; Fat, 15.0 grams.
Calories, 262 per serving.

Princess Loaf

3 cups Vege-Burger (see p. 174)
1 cup rice, cooked
½ cup onions, chopped and braised
1 cup almonds, roasted, chopped

5 eggs
1 cup half-and-half cream
¼ cup parsley, chopped
1 teaspoon Vegex (see p. 174)

1. Mix all ingredients well.
2. Pour in oiled pan.
3. Bake in 350°F oven for 1 hour and 15 minutes.
4. Serve with Brown Gravy (see p. 175).

Yield: 10 servings.

Carbohydrate, 19.5 grams; Protein, 9.4 grams; Fat, 11.0 grams.
Calories, 215 per serving.

Shepherd Pot Pie

1 cup potatoes, diced
½ cup celery, diced
½ cup onions, diced
1 carrot, diced
2 tablespoons margarine
¼ teaspoon salt
½ teaspoon Vejex (see p. 174)
½ tablespoon chicken-flavor seasoning (see p. 174)

4 tablespoons tomato soup
Hot water to cover vegetables
2⅓ ounces Vegetarian Skallops, cut in ½ inch squares, or 10 ounces of Prime roll (see p. 174)
1 tablespoon oil
½ tablespoon brewers' yeast
1 tablespoon cornstarch
1½ cups mashed potatoes

1. Cook first 10 ingredients.
2. Braise Skallops in oil and brewers' yeast. Add to mixture.
3. Dissolve cornstarch in a little water.
4. Place stew in shallow pan.
5. Using a pastry bag, flute the stew with mashed potatoes.
6. Sprinkle a little margarine over potatoes, and brown in 370°F oven.

Yield: 8 servings.

Carbohydrate, 28.0 grams; Protein, 7.0 grams; Fat, 15.0 grams.
Calories, 275 per serving.

Stroganoff with Noodles or Rice

1 pound Vegetable Steaks, cut in ½ and sliced very thin (see p. 174)
2 cups milk and juice of Steaks
1 tablespoon brewers' yeast
1 tablespoon of margarine
6 ounces mushroom slices
2 tablespoons flour
¼ cup onions, chopped and braised
¼ cup green onions, chopped and braised
¼ cup celery, chopped and braised
¼ cup peas or chopped parsley
2 teaspoons chicken-like seasoning (see p. 174)
½ teaspoon salt
1 tablespoon diced pimento
⅔ cup sour cream

1. Braise mushrooms in margarine.
2. Add flour, stir in milk and Steaks juice.
3. Braise Steaks in oil and brewers' yeast.
4. Add remaining ingredients, and heat.
5. Serve on hot cooked noodles or rice.

Yield: 10 servings.

Carbohydrate, 19.0 grams; Portein, 11.0 grams; Fat, 13.0 grams.
Calories, 237 per serving.

Soy-Cheese Patties

2 tablespoons green onions, minced
2 tablespoons oil
1 cup tofu, mashed
¼ cup breading meal or Special K flakes
¼ teaspoon lemon juice
2 tablespoons dry, instant, mashed potatoes
¼ cup milk
2 tablespoon walnuts, chopped

1. Place the oil and onions in a saucepan, and simmer until onions are soft but not brown.
2. Mash the tofu with a fork.
3. Add the milk to the tofu, then add the breading meal and nuts. Mix well.
4. Add the onion and oil mixture.
5. Add the instant, dry, mashed potatoes and the lemon juice.
6. Mix thoroughly.
7. Form into patties.
8. Roll in very fine flakes or breading meal.
9. Place on an oiled sheet, and bake at 350°F for about ½ hour or until nicely browned.

Yield: 4 patties.

Carbohydrate, 13.5 grams; Protein, 10.0 grams; Fat, 12.8 grams.
Calories, 207 per serving.

Soy-Cheese Scallops

½ pound tofu
½ cup scrambled eggs
½ cup mayonnaise
¼ cup parsley, chopped
1 tablespoon pimento, chopped

1 cup onions, chopped and braised
1 tablespoon Vegex (see p. 174)
2 cups cornflake crumbs
1 quart oil for frying

1. Steam tofu in double boiler ½ hour.
2. Drain and let it stand overnight.
3. Mash tofu and scrambled eggs.
4. Mix all ingredients and ½ of cornflake crumbs.
5. Make balls.
6. Roll in remaining cornflake crumbs.
7. Heat oil in deep pot to 350°F.
8. Deep fry the tofu balls to light brown.
9. Put in baking pan, and heat 20 minutes in 300°F oven.
10. Serve with Tartar Sauce (see p. 150).

Yield: 10 servings.

Carbohydrate, 9.6 grams; Protein, 10.0 grams; Fat, 6.9 grams.
Calories, 137 per serving.

Spanish Casserole

1 can 3-bean mix (2 cups)
2 onions, finely chopped
1 small green pepper
2 tablespoons margarine
1½ cups tomato puree
1 small can mushrooms

1 teaspoon Marmite or Savorex (see p. 174)
1 garlic clove, crushed
½ cup slivered almonds, toasted
½ cup fresh bread crumbs
¼ cup cream cheese

1. Sauté the onion, green pepper, and garlic in margarine.
2. Add the bean mix, tomato puree, and Marmite.
3. Puree mushrooms and half of the almonds, and reserve half the nuts to sprinkle on top.
4. Combine bread crumbs and cream cheese.
5. Add remainder of almonds, sprinkling on top of casserole.
6. Bake in moderate oven for 20 minutes just prior to serving.

Yield: 10 servings.

Carbohydrate, 20.0 grams; Protein, 6.5 grams; Fat, 9.8 grams.
Calories, 194 per serving.

Spinach Puff

¼ cup margarine
1½ tablespoons flour
2 cups cottage cheese
8 ounces frozen spinach, chopped
½ teaspoon salt
4 eggs, beaten
2 egg whites
1¾ cups white sauce, medium (see p. 175)

1. Melt margarine. Blend in flour.
2. Add cottage cheese gradually. Blend.
3. Add spinach and mix well.
4. Cool slightly.
5. Stir in salt and beaten eggs.
6. Beat egg whites until stiff, and fold in.
7. Pour into baking pan.
8. Set in shallow pan of water.
9. Bake at 350°F for 30 minutes or until set.
10. Serve with white sauce.

Yield: 10 servings.

Carbohydrate, 7.9 grams; Protein, 11.7 grams; Fat, 10.3 grams.
Calories, 173 per serving.

Stuffed Cabbage

2 cups Vegetable Skallops (see p. 174)
½ cup onions, chopped and braised
1 tablespoon brewers' yeast
1 teaspoon paprika
1 teaspoon chili powder
2 eggs
4 cups tomato sauce
10 cabbage leaves
¼ cup oil

1. Steam cabbage leaves until tender.
2. Grind Skallops coarsely.
3. Braise Skallops in oil, and sprinkle with brewers' yeast.
4. Mix Skallops, eggs, onions, and seasonings.
5. Cut stems of cabbage. Spoon Skallops mixture onto cabbage leaves.
6. Roll the stuffed cabbage like enchiladas.
7. Fold in ends of cabbage leaves.
8. Place in greased pan, and pour tomato sauce on the cabbage.
9. Bake at 325°F for 20–25 minutes.

Yield: 10 servings.

Carbohydrate, 17.0 grams; Protein, 10.0 grams; Fat, 2.0 grams.
Calories, 128 per serving.

Tacos

12 tortillas	½ cup onions, chopped and braised
3 cups Vegetable Skallops (see p. 174)	1 tablespoon brewers' yeast
	⅓ cup oil
¼ cup catsup	1 cup lettuce, chopped
1 tablespoon chili	1 cup tomatoes, diced
1 teaspoon paprika	1 cup American cheese, shredded

1. Grind the Skallops, coarsely.
2. Braise Skallops and brewers' yeast in a little oil.
3. Mix Skallops, catsup, chili, paprika, and onions.
4. Spoon the Skallops mixture on tortillas. Fold each tortilla in half.
5. Fry each taco on both sides in a little oil.
6. Mix lettuce, tomato, and cheese.
7. Open each taco, and put mixture of lettuce, tomato, and cheese on it, and serve. Add freshly chopped onions if desired.

Yield: 12 servings.

Carbohydrate, 12.0 grams; Protein, 12.0 grams; Fat, 9.0 grams.
Calories, 178 per serving.

Tamale Bake

¼ cup onions, chopped	½ cup cornmeal
3 tablespoons plus 2 teaspoons margarine	½ cup low-fat milk
	½ cup small curd cottage cheese
1½ cups chili bean soup	1 cup jack cheese, shredded
1¼ cups tomatoes, diced	¼ teaspoon salt
1½ cups whole kernel corn, frozen	

1. Sauté onions in melted margarine.
2. Add chili bean soup, tomatoes, and corn.
3. Heat to boiling.
4. Remove from heat.
5. Blend cornmeal with low-fat milk and salt. Mix in cottage cheese.
6. Stir into chili mixture.
7. Spread into well-greased pan.
8. Bake at 350°F for 1 hour, or until firm.
9. Top with jack cheese.
10. Bake at 325°F for 5 minutes to melt cheese.

Yield: 10 servings.

Carbohydrate, 28.9 grams; Protein, 7.0 grams; Fat, 3.3 grams.
Calories, 170 per serving.

Tofu Balls or Cutlets

3¼ cups tofu
3 eggs
1 teaspoon yeast extract
¼ cup onions, chopped
⅓ cup mayonnaise

2½ teaspoons red pepper, diced
2 teaspoons parsley sprigs, chopped
½ teaspoon chicken-like seasoning
(see p. 174)
1 cup cornflake crumbs

1. Place all ingredients in mixing bowl except cornflake crumbs. Mix well.
2. Shape mixture into 20 small balls.
3. Roll each ball in cornflake crumbs.
4. Deep-fat fry balls to a golden brown.
5. If cutlets are desired, take same mixture as used to make balls, press flat to make 10 cutlets, put on a greased baking pan, and bake for 20–25 minutes at 350°F.

Yield: 10 servings.

Carbohydrate, 9.6 grams; Protein, 10.0 grams; Fat, 6.9 grams. Calories, 137 per serving.

Tofu Balls with Tartar Sauce

2 cups tofu
1 egg, scrambled
½ cup cornflake crumbs
2 tablespoons onions, chopped
¼ teaspoon salt

¼ teaspoon torumel yeast
1 tablespoon plus 1 teaspoon mayonnaise
1 tablespoon red pepper, diced
1 teaspoon chicken-like seasoning
(see p. 174)

1. Steam tofu for 30 minutes. Refrigerate.
2. Grind tofu and scrambled egg.
3. Place all ingredients in mixing bowl. Mix well.
4. Form mixture into 20 balls, and roll each ball in cornflake crumbs.
5. Deep-fry the tofu balls at 375°F to a golden brown, approximately 3 minutes.
6. Place tofu balls in oven. Bake at 250°F for 20 minutes.

Note: May be served with Tartar Sauce (see p. 150).

Yield: 10 servings (2 balls each).

Carbohydrate, 12.0 grams; Protein, 9.0 grams; Fat, 11.0 grams. Calories, 180 per serving.

Vege-Burger Mix Deluxe

2¼ cups Vege-Burger (see
  p. 174)
½ cup walnuts, chopped
¾ cup rolled oats
2 tablespoons cream cheese
3 eggs
½ cup onions

2 tablespoons margarine
½ teaspoon garlic powder
¾ teaspoon chili powder
½ teaspoon salt
½ teaspoon sage
¾ cup bread crumbs

1. Place first four ingredients in mixing bowl, and mix thoroughly.
2. Sauté onions in margarine, then add to mixture.
3. Add remaining ingredients. Mix on medium speed for 10 minutes.
4. Fry patties in frypan until done.

Yield: 15 servings.

Carbohydrate, 5.5 grams; Protein, 9.9 grams; Fat, 7.8 grams.
Calories, 131 per serving.

Tofu with Mushroom Sauce

2 cups small-cubed tofu
2 tablespoons oil
¼ cup diced mushrooms
1 package (2 envelopes)
  Gravy Quik (see p. 174)

1 bunch green onions
2 stems celery, finely cut
½ tablespoon soy sauce
2 cups cold water

1. Place onions, oil, celery, and mushrooms in saucepan.
2. Sauté until vegetables are soft, but do not brown.
3. Add soy sauce.
4. Dissolve Gravy Quik in cold water.
5. Cook until thick.
6. Add cooked Gravy Quik to the vegetable mixture.
7. Place the cubed tofu in a flat baking dish.
8. Cover with gravy-vegetable mixture.
9. Let stand for 1 to 2 hours or overnight to allow tofu to become well-seasoned.
10. Bake in 350°F oven for 45 minutes.

Yield: 4 ½-cup servings.

Carbohydrate, 6.9 grams; Protein, 8.0 grams; Fat, 12.0 grams.
Calories, 179 per serving.

Tofu and Brown Rice Casserole

2½ teaspoons oil
1½ onions, thinly sliced
1 cup cooked brown rice
1½ cups tofu, steamed
1 teaspoon salt

1 cup milk
¼ to ½ cup bread crumbs
2 ounces yellow cheese, grated
¼ cup Parmesan cheese

1. Preheat oven to 350°F.
2. In a large, hot skillet, coated with 2 teaspoons of oil, add onions, and sauté until lightly browned.
3. Add brown rice, then tofu, sautéing each for 2 minutes.
4. Season with salt.
5. Place tofu and onion mixture in casserole.
6. Pour in milk, then sprinkle with bread crumbs and cheeses.
7. Bake for about 15 to 20 minutes at 350°F, or until cheese is nicely brown.

Yield: 8 servings.

Carbohydrate, 17.7 grams; Protein, 10.9 grams; Fat, 10.3 grams.
Calories, 208 per serving.

Vegetable Stew

2 pounds plus 6 ounces Vegetarian Skallops, approximately 4½ cups (see p. 174)
1½ tablespoons brewers' yeast
3 tablespoons oil
1 medium potato, cubed
⅔ cup celery, diced

1 cup onions, chopped
1 cup carrots, diced
1 cup peas, frozen
½ cup tomato soup
1½ teaspoons chicken-like seasoning (see p. 174)
1½ teaspoons salt
¾ cup cornstarch
⅓ cup plus 1 tablespoon water

1. Braise Skallops in oil, and sprinkle with yeast.
2. Combine cornstarch and water. Mix well.
3. Combine all other ingredients. Add cornstarch mixture.
4. Cook until all vegetables are tender.

Yield: 10 servings.

Carbohydrate, 21.2 grams; Protein, 12.3 grams; Fat, 6.6 grams.
Calories, 192 per serving.

Tastee Cuts Deluxe

10 Tastee Cuts (see p. 174)
1 cup onions, chopped and braised
1 cup canned mushrooms
2 cups sour cream

4 cups liquid prepared by mixing ½ milk with ½ mushroom juice
1 tablespoon cornstarch
1 teaspoon salt
2 cups bread crumbs

1. Dip Tastee Cuts in batter, and roll each in the bread crumbs.
2. Fry in a little oil.
3. Heat milk and thicken with cornstarch dissolved in a little water.
4. Mix milk mixture, mushrooms, onions, sour cream, and seasoning.
5. Place Tastee Cuts in pan, and pour the milk mixture over the steaks.
6. Bake in 350°F oven for 20 to 25 minutes.

Batter

1 cup milk, warm
1 teaspoon Vejex (see p. 174)
½ teaspoon salt

2 tablespoons flour
2 eggs

1. Mix first three ingredients well.
2. Add flour, and mix until smooth.
3. Add eggs. Mix well.

Yield: 10 servings.

Carbohydrate, 21.0 grams; Protein, 16.0 grams; Fat, 5.9 grams.
Calories, 204 per serving.

Vegetarian Salmon

1 cup onion, grated
6 ounces Nuteena (see p. 174)
3 eggs
1 teaspoon Marmite (see p. 174)
8 ounces carrots, grated

¾ cup cooked white rice
2 tablespoons margarine
1 cup tomato juice
1 cup milk
Salt to taste

1. Mash Nuteena and add beaten eggs.
2. Dissolve Marmite in milk.
3. Mix all ingredients together.
4. Pour into oiled casserole dish.
5. Bake at 350°F oven until set.

Yield: 8 servings.

Carbohydrate, 13.9 grams; Protein, 7.9 grams; Fat, 9.0 grams.
Calories, 169 per serving.

Vegetarian Patties with Brown Rice or Braised Onions

1 pound, 4 ounces Vege-
   Burger (see p. 174)
6 ounces Proteena, ground
   (see p. 174)

1 cup onions, braised
6 eggs
¼ cup catsup
1 cup cornflake crumbs

1. Combine all ingredients.
2. Make patties.
3. Place on oiled baking pan and bake in 350°F oven.
4. Serve with fried brown rice with Vega-Chicken Sauce or braised onions.

Vega-Chicken Sauce

1½ cups water, hot
2 tablespoons margarine
1 teaspoon chicken-like
   seasoning (see p. 174)

Salt to taste
1 tablespoon cornstarch

1. Combine all ingredients except cornstarch.
2. Bring to a boil.
3. Dissolve cornstarch in a little water, and use to thicken the mixture.

Yield: 12 servings.

Carbohydrate, 12.0 grams; Protein, 16.5 grams; Fat, 6.3 grams.
Calories, 168 per serving.

Walnut Loaf

1 cup onions, dehydrated
⅝ cup unflavored protein
   (textured vegetable protein,
   or Granburger, see p. 174)
2¼ cups water
1 tablespoon plus 1 teaspoon
   lemon juice
⅓ cup carrots, shredded
¾ cup celery, chopped

1 cup walnuts, chopped
7 eggs
2 cups low-fat milk
2 teaspoons parsley
1 teaspoon salt
⅜ teaspoon sage
2 tablespoons beef-like seasoning
   (see p. 174)

1. Reconstitute the onions and protein in boiling water.
2. Add the lemon juice and shredded carrots immediately.
3. Place the remaining ingredients in mixing bowl, add the onion/burger mixture, and mix.
4. Pour into loaf pan. Bake at 350°F for 45 minutes or until done.

Yield: 10 servings.

Carbohydrate, 35.0 grams; Protein, 12.8 grams; Fat, 19.4 grams.
Calories, 366 per serving.

Walnut Patties

1½ cups roasted almonds, coarsely chopped
1½ cups Vege-Burger (see p. 174)
½ cup onions, chopped and braised
6 eggs
1 cup half-and-half cream
1 teaspoon salt
1 cup bread crumbs
½ cup parsley, chopped

1. Mix all ingredients.
2. Make into patties.
3. Place patties on oiled baking pan.
4. Bake in 300°F oven for 20 to 25 minutes.

Note: May serve with Brown Gravy (see p. 175).
Yield: 10 servings.

Carbohydrate, 13.5 grams; Protein, 14.7 grams; Fat, 15.0 grams.
Calories, 248 per serving.

Western Stew with Biscuits

1 cup carrots, coarsely diced
1 cup celery, coarsely diced
1 cup onions, coarsely diced
1 cup potatoes, coarsely diced
1 cup peas
½ pound margarine
2 cups tomato soup
1 tablespoon chicken-like seasoning (see p. 174)
1 teaspoon salt
3 cups water
1½ pounds Prime, diced (see p. 174)
½ cup cornstarch

1. Cook all vegetables in water except peas.
2. When done, mix cornstarch in water to a buttermilk thickness.
3. Thicken stew, and add Prime, peas, tomato soup, and seasonings.
4. Serve with biscuits.

Yield: 10 servings.

Carbohydrate, 30.0 grams; Protein, 8.0 grams; Fat, 10.0 grams.
Calories, 242 per serving.

Zucchini Casserole

1½ pounds zucchini squash, sliced
1 can creamed corn
1 tablespoon melted margarine
1 small onion, chopped

1 small green pepper, chopped
2 eggs
Salt to taste
Italian herb seasoning to taste
¾ cup Cheddar cheese, shredded

1. Mix all ingredients well.
2. Put in greased casserole.
3. Place casserole in pan of water.
4. Bake at 350°F for 30 minutes.

Yield: 8 servings.

Carbohydrate, 12.0 grams; Protein, 5.7 grams; Fat, 6.1 grams.
Calories, 129 per serving.

Zucchini-Cheese Casserole

2 pounds zucchini squash, cut into ½-inch slices
½ cup boiling water
1 egg, lightly beaten
1 pound cottage cheese
1 cup cooked brown rice

1 onion, finely chopped
Salt to taste
½ teaspoon marjoram
1 tablespoon chives, chopped
¼ cup Parmesan cheese, grated

1. Place squash and boiling water in a saucepan. Cover and boil 5 minutes. Drain well.
2. Preheat oven to 350°F.
3. Combine the egg, cottage cheese, rice, onion, salt, marjoram, and chives.
4. Place half the squash in the bottom of a buttered casserole, top with half the rice mixture, then repeat layers.
5. Sprinkle with the Parmesan cheese, and bake 45 minutes at 350°F.

Yield: 8 servings.

Carbohydrae, 12.2 grams; Protein, 11.7 grams; Fat, 5.7 grams.
Calories, 147 per serving.

Zucchini Patties

4 cups zucchini squash,
  shredded
1½ cups cottage cheese
1 cup bread crumbs

7 eggs
1 teaspoon garlic powder
1 teaspoon salt

1. Mix all ingredients well.
2. Make ½ cup patties, and place on oiled baking sheet.
3. Bake in 325°F oven for 25 to 30 minutes.

Yield: 12 servings—1 pattie, ½ cup size.

Carbohydrate, 11.1 grams; Protein, 8.9 grams; Fat, 4.0 grams.
Calories, 116 per serving.

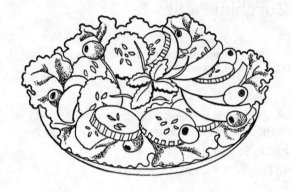

Garnish Your Foods

If it is true that "we eat with our eyes," how important is the *appearance* of food! A few minutes to consider those extra touches known as garnishes will be well spent. An artistic touch can take the humblest object and make it into a masterpiece of beauty. One needs to be beauty conscious to become a food artist, and make every meal a work of art.

Everyone can exercise creative ability, using decorative materials worthy of the dishes to be embellished. Accessories may be prepared ahead of time and added only at the last minute to insure freshness. The decor should fit the occasion and the dish itself, in taste and eye appeal, and of course in edibility and appetite appeal.

The artistic touch really consists of simplicity in design; such as, for example, arranging several spears of asparagus diagonally with tips crossed, or simply laying several spears parallel and crossing them with pimento strips. The true artist knows when to stop. The question isn't always what to add, sometimes it is what *not* to add.

Here are some questions to consider in garnishing:

1. Are the foods combined properly?
2. Are the foods prepared in a way that brings out the best and brightest natural color?
3. Are the foods arranged attractively on plates or serving dishes?
4. Is there variety of shapes?
5. Is there variety of textures?
6. Would some foods be better served in separate dishes?
7. Are the cold foods really cold, crisp, and bright?
8. Are the hot foods served hot and not overdone?

Beauty may be accentuated by using colorful dishes or decorations. There is a definite art in food color; art is important to those who willingly or reluctantly consume the food.

Each meal should be planned as though it were intended for a king or queen!

Fruits and vegetables may be used in many delightful ways. Following are a few ideas:

1. Apples
   a. Wedges, dipped in lemon juice to prevent discoloration.
   b. Slices, peeled and cut with a round cutter, the center emphasized with a cherry.
   c. Crab apples, used whole.
   d. Red apples, sliced, overlapping.
2. Asparagus tips in crisscross position.
3. Avocado slices with finely chopped parsley on outside edge.
4. Artichokes with red radish slices between the leaves.
5. Green beans cut in lozenges or arranged in little bundles.
6. Beets, waffle slices to top salad.
7. Broccoli, tiny bunches of intense green broccoli on top of tomato slice or as bouquet arrangement with other garnishes.
8. Carrot, curls, sticks, julienne, or cooked and cut in circles.
9. Cauliflower roses to place beside a green vegetable.
10. Celery leaves or curls to top a salad.
11. Cherry tomatoes stuffed with FriChik salad (see p. 174) or cottage cheese.
12. Cherries, canned, maraschino, to top whipped cream.
13. Chives, cooked or raw, cut or in long strips.
14. Colored coconut, sprinkled over a fruit cup.
15. Cream cheese, cut in shapes or placed around pears with leaf at top and cottage cheese in center.
16. Corn, tiny ears, canned, 3 small ears placed to the side of a salad.
17. Cucumbers, grooved with fork and sliced, or cut in shapes, overlapping 3 slices to one side.
18. Fruit kabobs on sticks to top fruit salads and some desserts.
19. Grapefruit flowers, made from grapefruit peel and colored, with red coloring. Peel by following a circular movement around grapefruit, making a continuous strip. Soak in color until desired color is obtained. Remove from color liquid, dry with paper towel, and arrange in shape of a rose.
20. Green mint leaves on cheese cake, honeydew melon, salad molds.
21. Mushrooms, heads stuffed, or slices. May be used with roasts, salads vegetables, or stuffed eggs.
22. Nuts, almond slices, and other nuts, in vegetables, or on salads or roasts.

23. Olives, black, stuffed, thinly sliced to top a salad or an entrée.
24. Onions, small, sliced, or with tomato slices and parsley.
25. Oranges, sliced, sectioned, or cubed to top a salad.
26. Parsley, sprig to one side of plate.
27. Peaches and pears, cut, diced, sliced, arranged with pimento.
28. Peppers, green, cut, diced, sliced, arranged with pimento.
29. Pimentos, red, cut in strips or shapes and arranged by entrée.
30. Pineapple, sliced, jullienne; canned or fresh, placed to one side of a vegetable.
31. Radishes, variety of flowers, accordions, slices, finely diced with red peel left on in which to roll balls of cheese.
32. Tomatoes, wedges, slices, diced, with other vegetables such as olives, pickles, peppers, in arrangements such as tomato wedge crossed with pickle topped with an olive.
33. Water cress, fresh only, with strawberries cut lengthwise, or with melon balls, grapefruit sections, and whole grapes.

Not to be overlooked are:

1. Molds made of cream cheese, gelatins, or fruits, and placed on large items such as roasts, loaves, and salads.
2. Stars of creamed cheese on red or green Jello.
3. Unique arrangements and designs.
4. Miniature items such as jelly roll on a fancy stick used for buffets or some desserts.

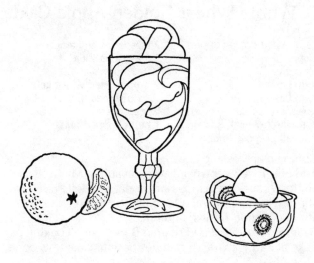

Not-Too-Sweet Desserts

Many desserts can be simple and nourishing. Fresh fruits, arranged in a bowl or on a platter, are always in "good taste." A simple crust or sponge torte to which fruit may be added—with simple glaze as a finishing touch—is attractive and delicious. A combination of fruits and nuts may be welcome. When fresh fruits are not available, frozen fruits may be used in the same manner.

Simple desserts may be not only nourishing but also not high in calories. Fruit pies are an example. Cakes using fruit as the sweetener are often used. Usually one can alter the amount of sugar in a recipe to decrease the total calories.

Desserts are meant to be enjoyed, but the dessert should be *simple*. Fruits lend themselves beautifully to the completion of a meal with something both dainty and tasty. Their nutrients consist chiefly of natural fruit sugars which are ready for immediate absorption.

There are more than 300 varieties of fruit from which to make choices. Some of the recipes in this book are low in calories but still very desirable. Most recipes have combined foods to increase their nutritive values.

Whole-Wheat Golden-Apple Cake

4 cups grated golden apples
2 eggs
½ cup oil
½ cup honey
½ cup brown sugar
1 teaspoon vanilla
1 cup whole-wheat flour
¼ cup all-purpose flour

2 teaspoons cinnamon
2 teaspoons soda
¼ teaspoon salt
¼ cup toasted wheat germ
½ cup shredded coconut
½ cup raisins
1 cup chopped nuts

1. Combine apples and eggs.
2. Add oil, honey, brown sugar, and vanilla. Mix well.
3. Sift together flours, cinnamon, soda, and salt.
4. Stir in wheat germ and add to apple mixture.
5. Stir in coconut, raisins, and nuts.
6. Pour into a greased and floured 9-by-14-inch baking pan.
7. Bake at 350°F about 30 minutes or until cake tests done.

Yield: 12 servings.

Carbohydrate, 44.5 grams; Protein, 6.5 grams; Fat, 18.4 grams.
Calories, 370 per serving.

Lemon-Pudding Cake

3 egg whites
6 tablespoons sugar
¾ cup flour
⅛ teaspoon salt
2 tablespoons melted
  margarine

4 tablespoons lemon juice
1 teaspoon grated lemon rind
3 egg yolks
1½ cups milk

1. Beat egg whites in casserole until foam holds its shape.
2. Sprinkle sugar, 2 tablespoons at a time, over foam, beating after each addition.
3. After final beating, mixture should be white, moist, and shiny.
4. Combine sugar, flour, salt, and margarine; add lemon juice and rind.
5. Add egg yolk and milk. Mix well.
6. Fold into beaten whites.
7. Set casserole in an inch of water and bake at 325°F for 45 minutes.

Yield: 6–8 servings.

Carbohydrate, 36.8 grams; Protein, 3.2 grams; Fat, 5.3 grams.
Calories, 204 per serving.

Orange-Crumble Cake
Cake

¼ cup plus 1½ teaspoons
  cake flour
½ cup margarine
½ cup cracker meal

¼ cup sugar
7 tablespoons coconut, shredded

Filling

1 cup orange juice
7¼ tablespoons sugar
2 tablespoons cornstarch

1 egg
1¼ teaspoons margarine

1. Mix Filling ingredients in double boiler.
2. Cook until thickened and clear. Set aside.
3. Mix well the Cake ingredients.
4. Grease pan, cover with ½ of Cake mixture.
5. Spread Filling mixture on top of Cake mixture.
6. Cover Filling mixture with rest of Cake mixture, sandwiching Filling mixture.
7. Pat down only by hand—not too hard.
8. Bake at 350°F until golden brown.

Yield: 8 servings.

Carbohydrate, 40.6 grams; Protein, 2.5 grams; Fat, 15.9 grams.
Calories, 315 per serving.

Chinese Almond Cookies

3 cups flour
1½ cups vegetable shortening
1 cup sugar
½ teaspoon baking soda

¼ teaspoon salt
1 tablespoon almond extract
1 large egg

1. Beat egg lightly.
2. Add gradually to all other ingredients.
3. Mix and knead until soft.
4. Form into balls about the size of a quarter and flatten with thumb.
5. Set ½ of a whole almond in center of cookie (almond may be soaked in red food coloring).
6. Bake approximately 20 minutes in a 350–375°F oven.

Yield: 4 dozen small cookies.

Carbohydrate, 9.4 grams; Protein, .9 gram; Fat, 7.1 grams.
Calories, 105 per cookie.

Coconut Macaroon Cookies

3 cups sugar
¼ cup cornstarch
¼ cup cake flour
1 teaspoon salt

6 tablespoons honey
1½ cups egg whites
3 cups macaroon coconut

1. Mix together the egg whites, sugar, flour, cornstarch, salt, and honey. Warm mixture in a double boiler.
2. Add macaroon coconut and beat well.
3. Drop onto a cookie sheet with a spoon.
4. Bake at 350°F until light golden brown.

Yield: 6 dozen.

Carbohydrate, 12.0 grams; Protein, .8 gram; Fat, .2 gram.
Calories, 55 per cookie.

Dream Bars

½ cup margarine
1 cup graham cracker crumbs
1 cup coconut

1 cup chocolate chips
1 cup pecans or walnuts, chopped
1 can condensed milk

1. Melt margarine in an 8-inch square baking pan.
2. Sprinkle dry ingredients over the margarine in the order listed.
3. Pour condensed milk over the top. *DO NOT STIR.*
4. Bake in 350°F oven for 30 minutes.
5. Cool before cutting into squares.

Yield: 2 dozen small cookies.

Carbohydrate, 16.0 grams; Protein, 2.3 grams; Fat, 11.2 grams.
Calories, 173 per cookie.

Apple Whip

½ cup milk, evaporated
1 cup applesauce

1 tablespoon lemon juice
Syrup to taste

1. Chill milk thoroughly, then whip until stiff.
2. Fold in the cold applesauce and lemon juice.
3. Sweeten with syrup.
4. Sprinkle with nutmeg, if desired.

Yield: 3 servings; *serving:* ½ cup.

Carbohydrate, 26.0 grams; Protein, 4.3 grams; Fat, .3 gram.
Calories, 122 per serving.

Note: This mixture may be poured into a refrigerator tray and frozen.

Date-Swirl Cookies

1¼ cups sugar
½ cup vegetable shortening
½ (scant) teaspoon baking
  powder
½ teaspoon vanilla
2 eggs
½ teaspoon salt
¾ cup plus 1 tablespoon milk
5 cups cake flour
2 cups chopped dates
1 teaspoon sugar
Water as needed

1. Cream sugar and shortening.
2. Add eggs and vanilla. Beat mixture well.
3. Sift flour, salt, and baking powder together, then add alternately with milk to mixture.
4. Chill while fixing date filling.
5. To make date filling, grind dates, then add 1 teaspoon sugar and water to make a spreadable paste.
6. Roll out dough and spread with filling. Roll up like a jelly roll.
7. Cut into slices and bake at 350°F (approximately 10 minutes or until delicately brown).

Yield: 5 dozen.

Carbohydrate, 37.9 grams; Protein, 2.6 grams; Fat, 6.2 grams.
Calories, 214 per 2 cookies.

Wheat-Germ Cookies

⅔ cup vegetable shortening
2 tablespoons molasses
½ teaspoon salt
½ cup brown sugar, firmly
  packed
2 eggs, well beaten
1 cup chopped nuts (pecans,
  walnuts)
1½ cups seedless raisins
1 cup wheat germ
1 cup oatmeal, quick-cooking
1½ cups sifted all-purpose flour (or
  whole-wheat flour)
1 teaspoon vanilla

1. Cream shortening, salt, and molasses together.
2. Add sugar gradually. Cream until light.
3. Add beaten eggs and mix well.
4. Add raisins, nuts, wheat germ, and oatmeal. Mix.
5. Add vanilla and flour. Mix lightly.
6. Drop from spoon onto oiled baking sheet.
7. Bake at 375°F for 15–20 minutes until delicate brown.

Yield: 4 dozen.

Carbohydrate, 11.7 grams; Protein, 1.9 grams; Fat, 2.2 grams.
Calories, 74 per cookie.

Baked Apples

4 baking apples
¼ cup honey

½ cup water
1 teaspoon grated lemon or orange rind

1. Preheat oven to 375°F.
2. Wash and core apples and place in baking dish.
3. Combine honey with the water and grated rind.
4. Pour over the apples and bake, covered, for 30 minutes. Baste 2 or 3 times.
5. Uncover, baste again, and bake 15 minutes longer or until tender.

Yield: 4 servings.

Carbohydrate, 38.1 grams; Protein, .4 gram; Fat, .9 gram.
Calories, 162 per serving.

Apricot Whip

2 8-ounce cans apricot halves, dietetic pack
1 envelope (4-serving size), orange D-Zerta gelatin

1 cup boiling water
1 tablespoon lemon juice

1. Drain apricots. Measure apricot liquid, then add water to make 1 cup.
2. Chop apricots and set aside.
3. Dissolve gelatin in boiling water.
4. Add measured liquid and lemon juice.
5. Chill until slightly thickened.
6. Then place in bowl of ice water; whip with rotary beater until fluffy and thick.
7. Fold in chopped apricots.
8. Pour into 6 individual molds.
9. Chill until firm.

Yield: 4 servings; *serving:* ¾ cup.

Carbohydrate, 12.4 grams; Protein, .6 gram; Fat, 0 gram.
Calories, 52 per serving.

Banana Custard

½ cup whole milk   3 drops vanilla
1 egg   ½ medium banana

1. Scald the milk, beat the egg slightly, and stir in the milk and vanilla.
2. Rinse 2 custard cups with cold water to prevent the custard from adhering to the sides.
3. Slice one fourth banana into each custard cup, and pour half the custard mixture over it.
4. Place the cups in a deep baking pan. Surround the cup with hot water.
5. Bake in a moderate oven until firm or until a knife blade inserted in the center of the custard comes out clean. Do not allow the water to boil because it might cause the custard to separate.
6. Serve by removing the custard from the cup and putting it into a sherbet dish.

Yield: 2 servings; *serving:* ½ cup.

Carbohydrate, 10.6 grams; Protein, 5.9 grams; Fat, 5.0 grams.
Calories, 111 per serving.

Baked Maple Apples

8 large, tart apples   16 dates or 16 tablespoons raisins
½ cup maple syrup   2 teaspoons grated lemon rind

1. Pare top half of apples, remove cores.
2. Place apples in large baking dish.
3. Stuff each apple with 2 dates or 2 tablespoons of raisins.
4. Combine syrup with lemon rind and a little water.
5. Pour over apples, and bake at 375°F for 1 hour until tender.
6. Baste with syrup occasionally.
7. Serve warm or chilled.

Yield: 8 servings; *serving:* 1 apple.

Carbohydrate, 53.4 grams; Protein, .6 gram; Fat, .3 gram.
Calories, 219 per serving.

Banana Popsicle

8 dates
1 cup applesauce, unsweetened

½ cup coconut, unsweetened
8 bananas

1. Chop dates very fine.
2. Mix with applesauce.
3. Cover banana with date butter.
4. Roll in unsweetened coconut.
5. Place on flat pan and put in freezer. Let freeze overnight.

Yield: 8 servings.

Carbohydrate, 35.9 grams; Protein, 1.7 grams; Fat, 2.0 grams.
Calories, 169 per serving.

Bread Pudding

4½ cups whole milk
6 eggs
½ teaspoon salt
2 teaspoons vanilla

1¼ cups bread pieces prepared from approximately 2½ slices
¼ cup sugar

1. Beat eggs well.
2. Add salt, vanilla, sugar. Beat well.
3. Add milk. Beat well.
4. Put bread pieces in pan, and soak with custard mixture.
5. Bake for 45 minutes at 350°F, then cover with baking paper. Continue to bake until firm, about another 15–20 minutes.

Yield: 10 servings.

Carbohydrate, 11.2 grams; Protein, 10.8 grams; Fat, 9.8 grams.
Calories, 175 per serving.

Cranberry Pudding

3¼ cups cranberry juice
3 tablespoons instant tapioca

3 tablespoons sugar

1. Dissolve instant tapioca in small amount of cranberry juice.
2. Boil the rest of the cranberry juice.
3. After it has boiled, add tapioca mixture.
4. Add sugar, and stir well.

Yield: 6 servings.

Carbohydrate, 23.2 grams; Protein, 0 gram; Fat, 0 gram.
Calories, 93 per serving.

Egg Custard

1 quart milk
¼ cup sugar
10 eggs, beaten

Pinch salt
½ teaspoon vanilla

1. Mix all ingredients together. Blend well.
2. Pour mixture into 10 individual custard cups that have been rinsed under tap water.
3. Bake in a pan of water at 325°F until firm (about 1 hour).

Yield: 10 servings.

Carbohydrate, 10.2 grams; Protein, 10.4 grams; Fat, 9.6 grams. Calories, 169 per serving.

Note: A casserole may be used instead of the cups.

Fresh Fruit Cup

1½ cups fresh strawberries
1½ cups fresh pineapple
1½ cups fresh honeydew
  melon balls
½ cup fresh orange juice

1 tablespoon fresh lemon juice
2 tablespoons vanilla
6 sprigs of mint

1. Wash and hull berries.
2. Dice pineapple, and combine with berries and melon balls.
3. Combine orange juice, lemon juice, and vanilla, then pour over fruit.
4. Toss lightly once or twice. Place in sherbet glasses with sprig of fresh mint.
5. Serve very cold.

Yield: 6 servings.

Carbohydrate, 12.6 grams; Protein, .8 gram; Fat, .4 gram. Calories, 57 per serving.

Fruited Barley

1 cup barley
1 teaspoon salt

1½ cups dried fruit: raisins or prunes
  or peaches or apricots
2 tablespoons lemon juice (if desired)

1. Soak barley in water for 12 hours.
2. Add salt and fruit. Cook 1 hour or until barley is soft.
3. Before serving, add brown sugar and lemon juice.
4. Serve warm.

Yield: 8 servings; *serving:* 1 cup.

Carbohydrate, 39.8 grams; Protein, 4.2 grams; Fat, .7 gram. Calories, 183 per serving.

Fruit Tapioca

1 tablespoon tapioca, quick cooking
½ cup fruit juice

1. Place tapioca in pan with fruit juice. Stir well. Cherry, grape, and plum juice are most outstanding in flavor. Allow to boil over low heat.
2. After boiling 1 or 2 minutes, remove from heat and cool before serving.
3. Garnish with pieces of fruit.

Yield: 1 serving; *serving:* ½ cup.

Carbohydrate, 16.0 grams; Protein, 1.8 grams; Fat, .9 gram.
Calories, 79 per serving.

Indian Pudding

¼ cup corn meal
2 cups hot non-fat milk
¼ cup sugar
⅛ teaspoon baking soda
½ teaspoon salt
½ teaspoon ground ginger
½ teaspoon ground cinnamon
¼ cup molasses
1 cup cold non-fat milk
Dash nutmeg

1. Preheat oven to 275°F.
2. Stir the cornmeal, a little at a time, into the hot milk. Cook over low heat, or in double boiler, stirring constantly, for 15 minutes or until thick. Remove from heat.
3. Mix together the sugar, soda, salt, and spices. Stir into the cornmeal mixture.
4. Thoroughly mix in the molasses and cold milk.
5. Pour into a 1-quart casserole and bake 2 hours.
6. Serve warm with light sprinkling of nutmeg.

Yield: 8 servings.

Carbohydrate, 19.9 grams; Protein, 3.6 grams; Fat, .2 gram.
Calories, 96 per serving.

Orange Sauce

½ cup sugar
1 tablespoon cornstarch
Dash salt
Dash cinnamon
¾ cup boiling water

1 tablespoon oil
¼ cup orange juice
1 teaspoon grated orange rind
2 teaspoons lemon juice

1. In a saucepan, mix together the sugar, cornstarch, salt, and cinnamon.
2. Gradually add the water. Bring to a boil over medium heat, and cook, stirring, for 5 minutes.
3. Remove from heat. Add oil, orange and lemon juices, then the rind.
4. Serve over rice pudding, plain cake, or gingerbread.

Yield: 1 cup; serving: 1 tablespoon.

Carbohydrate, 7.1 grams; Protein, 0 gram; Fat, .9 gram.
Calories, 37 per serving.

Peaches with Meringue

6 medium peach halves, canned
1 tablespoon brown sugar
1 tablespoon lemon rind, grated

1 egg white, beaten
2 tablespoons sugar

1. Drain canned peaches and place six halves on oven-proof platter, hollow side up.
2. Sprinkle halves with brown sugar and lemon rind.
3. Make a meringue of egg white and 2 tablespoons sugar.
4. Spoon meringue on peach halves in peaks.
5. Broil or bake until peaches are heated through and meringue is delicately browned.
6. A dash of nutmeg or mace may be used in place of the lemon rind.

Yield: 6 servings; serving: ½ peach.

Carbohydrate, 11.7 grams; Protein, 1.3 grams; Fat, .1 gram.
Calories, 52 per serving.

Peanut Butter Candy

2 tablespoons peanut butter
2 tablespoons milk
2 tablespoons raisins

1 graham cracker
1 teaspoon vanilla

1. Cream peanut butter until smooth. Add 1 tablespoon milk, and mix until well blended.
2. Add the raisins and mix well.
3. Break one graham cracker into small pieces. Mix with peanut butter mixture.
4. Add 1 tablespoon of milk and vanilla.
5. Form into balls or make one bar-shaped piece.

Yield: 6 servings; *serving:* 1 ball.

Carbohydrate, 14.7 grams; Protein, 5.1 grams; Fat, 7.8 grams.
Calories, 149 per serving.

Baked Prune Whip

2 cups cooked prunes
4 tablespoons sugar
2 tablespoons orange juice

1 teaspoon grated orange peel
½ teaspoon cinnamon
4 egg whites

1. Preheat oven to 350°F.
2. Remove pits from the prunes, and puree in a blender.
3. Add 2 tablespoons of the sugar, orange juice, orange peel, and cinnamon. Blend well.
4. Beat the egg whites with the remaining 2 tablespoons of sugar until stiff.
5. Fold the pureed fruit into the egg whites, and pile lightly in a greased 1½ quart casserole.
6. Bake uncovered 20 to 30 minutes, until lightly browned and puffed up like a soufflé.
7. If desired, serve with Orange Sauce (see p. 231).

Yield: 8 servings.

Carbohydrate, 23.3 grams; Protein, 2.3 grams; Fat, trace.
Calories, 102 per serving.

Raspberry Bavarian

1 3-ounce package raspberry gelatin
1 cup boiling water
¾ cup cold water
3 tablespoons lemon juice

¾ cup raspberries, red, frozen, thawed, drained
3 tablespoons non-fat dry milk, instant
3 tablespoons ice-cold water

1. Thaw frozen raspberries.
2. Dissolve gelatin in the boiling water. Add cold water and lemon juice.
3. Refrigerate until mixture begins to thicken.
4. Drain the raspberries, reserving the juice to add just before serving.
5. Beat the non-fat dry milk with ice-cold water until consistency of whipped cream.
6. Beat gelatin until frothy.
7. Fold whipped milk into gelatin. Add the drained raspberries carefully.
8. Spoon into 6 sherbet glasses, chill, and add 1 tablespoon of reserved raspberry juice to each serving.

Yield: 6 servings; *serving:* 1 cup.

Carbohydrate, 17.8 grams; Protein, 2.5 grams; Fat, 1.0 gram.
Calories, 90 per serving.

Raspberry Parfait

1 tablespoon tapioca, instant
1 cup milk
1 egg
¼ teaspoon vanilla

⅛ teaspoon salt
1 cup raspberries
1 tablespoon whipped cream

1. Cook the tapioca and milk in a double boiler until tapioca becomes transparent.
2. Separate the egg yolk from the egg white, and beat the egg yolk.
3. Add the milk and tapioca mixture to the egg yolk, and return to the double boiler.
4. Cook until the mixture becomes thick, stirring frequently.
5. Cool slightly and then add the vanilla, salt, and raspberries.
6. Beat the egg white until stiff, then fold into the tapioca mixture.
7. Chill. Serve in parfait glasses. Top with whipped cream.

Yield: 4 servings; *serving:* ½ cup.

Carbohydrate, 16.7 grams; Protein, 9.4 grams; Fat, 9.6 grams.
Calories, 191 per serving.

Raspberry Razzle

1 cup raspberries, frozen, thawed
½ cup raspberry gelatin
¾ cup water, boiling
2 cups yogurt, plain
1 cup whipping cream

1. Drain raspberries, saving syrup.
2. Dissolve gelatin in syrup and boiling water.
3. Cool gelatin.
4. Blend in yogurt.
5. Whip cream stiff, then blend into gelatin mixture. Fold in raspberries.
6. Fill two pie shells. Chill until firm.
7. Garnish with whipped cream.

Yield: 12 servings.

Carbohydrate, 16.0 grams; Protein, 3.0 grams; Fat, 7.0 grams.
Calories, 136 per serving.

Rice Pudding

2 cups skim milk
3 tablespoons long-grain rice, raw
3 tablespoons sugar
¼ teaspoon salt
½ teaspoon vanilla extract
⅛ teaspoon nutmeg
⅛ teaspoon cinnamon
¼ cup light or dark seedless raisins

1. Preheat oven to 325°F.
2. Mix all ingredients together, and place in a 1-quart ovenproof casserole.
3. Bake uncovered for 2 to 2¼ hours or until rice is tender, occasionally stirring the surface skin into the pudding.
4. Serve warm or cold. If served cold, stir in enough skim milk to thin the pudding to desired consistency.

Yield: 6 servings.

Carbohydrate, 20.0 grams; Protein, 3.6 grams; Fat, .1 gram.
Calories, 95 per serving.

Strawberry Frozen Dessert

1 10-ounce package frozen strawberries
3 tablespoons frozen lemonade concentrate
6 tablespoons sugar
1½ cups evaporated skim milk
1 egg white
1 9-inch meringue shell (optional)

1. Combine the strawberries with the lemonade concentrate.
2. Pour the evaporated skim milk into a freezing tray, and freeze until mushy around the edges.
3. Put into a chilled bowl and beat to the consistency of whipped cream.
4. Beat 1 egg white until frothy. Add the sugar slowly, beating well after each addition.
5. Fold in the whipped milk and the strawberry mixture.
6. Pour into 3 freezing trays and freeze partially.
7. Place in a chilled bowl and beat again.
8. Return to the freezer for 8 hours or overnight.
9. Beat again until the dessert is the consistency of ice cream, and return to freezer.
10. Serve plain or in a meringue shell.

Yield: 9 servings.

Carbohydrate, 24.0 grams; Protein, 3.5 grams; Fat, .4 gram.
Calories, 110 per serving; 170 with meringue.

Yogurt Cheesecake

1 8-ounce package cream cheese
3 tablespoons honey
1 8-ounce carton unflavored yogurt

1. Beat the cream cheese with honey until fluffy.
2. Gradually mix in the yogurt until smooth.
3. Turn into prepared crust and spread evenly. Cover and refrigerate overnight or freeze.
4. Top with berries or Date-Nut Topping, if desired.

Date-Nut Topping

½ cup firmly packed, pitted dates, finely chopped
½ cup sliced or slivered almonds, coarsely chopped

1. Mix dates and almonds.
2. Sprinkle over cheesecake before serving.

Yield: 10 servings.

Filling:
Carbohydrate, 6.6 grams; Protein, 2.5 grams; Fat, 9.3 grams.
Calories, 120 per serving.

Topping:
Carbohydrate, 7.9 grams; Protein, 1.6 grams; Fat, 4.1 grams.
Calories, 75 per serving.

Index of Recipes